Group Process for the Health Professions

Group Process
for the
Health Professions

Second Edition

Edward E. Sampson, Ph.D.

Professor of Sociology
Adjunct Professor of Psychology
Clark University
Worcester, Massachusetts

Marya Marthas, R.N., Ed.D.

Lecturer
Department of Nursing
San Francisco State University
San Francisco, California
Psychologist
McLean Hospital
Belmont, Massachusetts

JOHN WILEY & SONS

New York • Chichester • Brisbane • Toronto • Singapore

Library of Congress Cataloging in Publication Data:

Sampson, Edward E.
  Group process for the health professions.
  (A Wiley medical publication)
  Bibliography: p.
  Includes index.
    1. Health care teams.   2. Small groups.
I. Marthas, Marya Sampson, joint author.
II. Title. [DNLM: 1. Group processes.
2. Interpersonal relations.   3. Physician-patient
relations.   W 62 S192g]
R729.5.H4S26   1981   302.3'02461   80-26487
ISBN 0-471-08279-1

Printed in the United States of America

10 9 8 7 6 5 4 3

Preface to the Second Edition

The goal that guided the first edition of this work remains intact in this revised version: to provide the health professional with the combined conceptual knowledge and practical skills needed to work effectively with small groups. As we noted in the first edition, the achievement of this goal builds on four critical foundations:

—Genuine care and concern for the group

—Knowledge of group process theories and concepts

—Development of the skills needed for effective intervention in a groups' ongoing process

—Sensitivity to one's self and to one's own impact as a participant-observer

Although we cannot teach the first of these four foundations, the remaining three have been woven into the fabric of this introductory text.

It is our hope that this revised edition retains the strengths of the original work even as we increase its usefulness by reorganizing and reorienting the manner of presentation. This edition, as we see it, does not demand a new base of materials for the health professional to learn; rather, what we seek in this revision is a more coherent and meaningful manner of organizing this fundamental base. To this end, therefore, we have reoriented the text by reorganizing its material into four units. Each is designed to focus on a different aspect of the subject.

Unit I lays a foundation for the need of group process in the health professions. Unit II introduces the key concepts involved in defining group process and in examining the central characteristics of groups. Unit III provides the essential theoretical background necessary to our understanding of group process. Unit IV directly confronts the applied issues, focusing on the concepts and skills of assessment and intervention.

The division into four units permits the reader to select any one unit for independent study. For example, it is possible to begin with Unit IV, focusing on the skills of assessment and intervention as a separate unit for study. Any unit permits this same kind of independent study. Needless to say, our own preference leans toward the eventual study of all four units and their many interconnections.

Reading a text, whatever its quality and manner of organization, can never substitute for actual "behind-the-wheel" practice. All we can hope to accomplish is to lay a solid foundation to guide and nourish that practice.

E.E.S.
M.M.

Contents

Group Process for the Health Professions

UNIT

I

Introduction

1. The Health Professional and Group Process
Group Process in Life and In Practice
Summary and Conclusions

No one would reasonably argue that the skills and techniques necessary to medical or nursing practice could be performed well without prior training and experience. We all recognize that certain special skills are required and that formal training is essential to gain those skills. However, when it comes to the area of group process, the story often takes a somewhat different twist. Here are some of the "resistances" and "reluctances" we have heard:

—Group process is basically intuitive and nonscientific knowledge; it is something that we instinctively know how to do well.

—Groups are frightening and confusing. They are beyond my own ability to understand and more than I could ever hope to work with.

—It is absurd to think that there are certain specific kinds of knowledge and skills that anyone could learn about group behavior; it is not at all like the material that I am used to in my other course work.

—Working with groups is an unnecessary frill; who really needs to know about groups in everyday practice?

In this opening unit, we address these questions and doubts. We lay a foundation for health professionals to develop knowledge and skills about group process. We base this on two major ideas:

1. The key role that groups play in human growth and development and in the maintenance or undermining of well-being makes it essential that anyone involved in health care gain an understanding and a reasonable level of skill in group process.
2. The role of groups in the everyday practice of the health professions warrants the practitioners' learning both about how groups function and how groups can function more effectively.

Thus, the study of group process is not an unnecessary frill that exists at some distant perimeter of medical or nursing practice. The knowledge and skills required to work effectively with groups are neither something intuitive or instinctive nor beyond anyone's ability to learn. There are definite skills and knowledge to be developed and learned, and there is an important place for group process in the repertoire of the health professionals' practice.

1

The Health Professional and Group Process

*H*uman beings are complicated creatures. We are biological organisms possessing qualities shared with all living systems and with others of our species. We are also psychological beings with distinctly human capabilities for thought, feeling, and reason. But that is not all. To say that we are also social, *group* beings is to recognize the complex web of interconnections that link us with other people. These links help define our *group character* and play a major role in our daily lives as well as our professional practice. It is difficult to imagine an activity in which our group character is not involved. The range within the health professions is broad: from simple conversations with patients and colleagues to meetings, rounds, conferences, training sessions, and so forth.

Nothing mysterious is intended in the reference to a person's group character. The concept directs our attention to two important issues. First, we usually conduct our practice within the actual presence of one or more other persons. And second, in light of this fact, we typically take them into account, adjusting our behavior to theirs, even as they adjust to ours. We and they thereby become participants in a group process. Our group character, therefore, refers to the bonds that connect us with others, a figurative line between persons representing the give-and-take adjustments each makes in the presence of the other.

Direct Connections

At times, these links are direct and relatively obvious:

Nurse Allen is obtaining intake information on her patient. She is preoccupied with asking questions and carefully recording the answers in their proper place on the many forms she must complete. The patient is anxious about this procedure. The more questions Nurse Allen asks, the greater the patient's anxiety becomes; soon, the anxiety interferes with her ability to hear the questions and even to think clearly enough to provide coherent answers. Nurse Allen has many other patients to deal with and so responds with growing annoyance to the patient's halting replies. She becomes more abrupt and demanding. The patient responds with even greater anxiety and difficulty in providing answers.

We do not want to belabor the obvious, but only to illustrate the bonds that link Nurse Allen and her patient, which give to each what we have called their group character.

What might appear to be a routine matter, obtaining intake information, involves an interpersonal process. The nurse's behavior is one element in that process; the patient's behavior, the other. Nurse Allen is not simply doing an interview to assess a patient on intake as a technician might assess a blood sample. Rather, she is involved as a participant in a process in which her behavior in conducting the interview affects the patient's response; in turn, the patient's responses affect the nurse's own behavior. Each is involved in adjusting her behavior to the behavior of the other person; this is the link that joins them.

In speaking of Nurse Allen's group character, we call attention to the idea that who she is is affected by who the other person is in the intake interview. Her character is that of someone who is annoyed and impatient. This is not a comment on her personality as much as on her manner of adjusting her behavior to the behavior of her patient. The patient likewise has a group character. Anxiety is not necessarily a quality she possesses separately from her reaction to Nurse Allen and the intake procedure. Each participant not only evokes a particular kind of response from the other but also responds to the other. We shall have more to say about this important matter and its practical implications in Chapters 2 and 3.

Subtle Connections

The links that relate us to others may also be subtle. We may participate in a group process with little awareness of the group character we are portraying.

The patient and his wife are about to leave the hospital; in her desire to reassure them that all is well, Dr. Welch tells the wife not to worry, that her husband's problem is only minor indigestion, and that nothing is really wrong. The couple begin to argue vehemently as they leave. Dr.

Welch turns around and continues with her other work, not realizing that her simple reassurance played a part in their family drama. Her assurance as a medical professional undercut the legitimacy of the husband's illness. Dr. Welch had defined him as not sick, never realizing that he had been using sickness as a way of avoiding responsibilities at home.

We are not suggesting that Dr. Welch should not have offered reassurance; we present this example to illustrate how the health professional may become a part of a group process without much awareness that this has even happened. In this case, Dr. Welch's behavior was less affected by others than it affected them; nevertheless, she became a member of that family's group process, if only for a brief moment. Obviously, knowledge of group process would help her in this type of intervention.

GROUP PROCESS IN LIFE AND IN PRACTICE

We have suggested several things regarding group process:

1. A person's life and professional practice involves other people.
2. People's group characters emerge as they interact with others.
3. Rarely if ever does a person practice without taking others into account, just as those others must act in the interpersonal context provided for them.
4. People may be participating in a group process even when they are unaware of that participation and even when "the group" includes only the individual and the patient or the individual and one other person.

This last point separates our approach to group process from some more traditional points of view. The traditional study of groups emphasizes something larger than the two-person (dyadic) transaction that we have used in our opening examples. Group and group process are thereby separated from the dyad and interpersonal process. Many of us have an intuitively larger context or longer-term relationship in mind when we speak of group process. The examples focus on small groups of two or three people; likewise, they examine relatively brief encounters.

Although we partly agree with these intuitive understandings and will even document the many distinctions in process that emerge when we move from the small dyadic encounter to include greater numbers of people (e.g., see Chapter 2), we are also suggesting that some important continuities exist between the study of interpersonal process and group process. The study of group process includes both of these groups as well as those more typically referred to as groups: that is, (1) relationships that have a relatively greater permanence and thus permit the development of relationships and structures, and (2) relationships that include larger numbers of people, encompassing patients as well as other people (e.g., colleagues, community groups, etc.). One point should be evident, we must seek to understand both group and interpersonal process and to develop as keen a sensitivity to our group character as we have of our biologic character.

It will be helpful to our understanding of group process in the health professions if we examine the wide variety of contexts, settings, and groups within which our practice tends to occur. We have outlined in Figure 1–1 some of the major areas of group participation relevant to the health professional. The point of all of this, quite simply, is to develop and expand group process training among health professionals. Our argument consists of two key ideas: (1) groups are central to human growth and development and play a continuing role in health maintenance or its absense; (2) groups are an important part of our daily practice.

The Role of Group Process in Human Growth and Development

The life history of human beings can be written in terms of the nature and types of groups in which they have been reared and in which they are involved. We are all born helpless and unable to function without support provided by other members of our species. Unlike many animals which achieve independence within a relatively brief

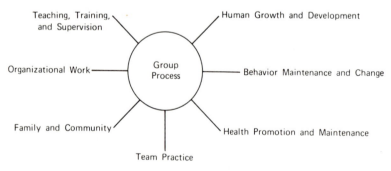

Figure 1-1. Group practice in life and in practice.

period after birth, the human infant must maintain a continued close dependence on others for a substantial period of its life. Even in adulthood, most people need others—the true hermit who can function independently of society is more myth than reality.

Primary Groups. Research suggests some of the serious consequences that face developing children who do not receive enough human interaction and contact. Sociologist C. H. Cooley (1909) early recognized the critical role that these *primary-group* contacts played in the emergence of social feelings and civilized persons. For Cooley, a primary group involves close, face-to-face associations of the sort found in the family, in play groups, and in many neighborhood and informal work groups. Such groups are characterized by their sense of "we" and "our" rather than the more individualistic "I" and "mine." These primary groups are the source of the person's emerging human social qualities; and for adults, they remain an important source of support and nurturance.

Although it has become fashionable to speculate on the breakdown of primary groups—e.g., neighborhood and friendship groups—in our modern society, research suggests the continuing importance and role of these groups in the life of the individual. Litwak and Szelenyi, for example (1969), determined where people would turn for help if they had a one-day stomachache, a two-week appendectomy, or a three-month broken leg. Their data suggested the importance of friendship and neighborhood groups for dealing with these and related types of health problems. In other words, even in our often impersonal modern urban society, people in trouble turn to primary groups for help and support.

The role of the primary group, especially the family, in health care has become increasingly relevant in the management of heart and cancer patients. The psychological impact of cancer, for example, has led health professionals to see the need to extend their treatment plans beyond the medical. The initial diagnosis, cancer, sets up a process that has a wide-ranging impact on patients and their families. Often, the initial shock gives way to anger, followed quickly by guilt and blame. The patient is angry but so too is the family, now threatened by the loss of one of its own. Patients and their families often blame themselves for their illness: "Perhaps we should have urged you to seek medical attention earlier; it's our fault." Fear is also a part of this process: "If my father has cancer, will I have an increased chance of getting it myself?"

The process we have briefly outlined is one that implicates the patients and their primary group; the management of the patient, therefore, must take that primary-group network into account as well. When the course of the disease is long-term, as tends to be the case with cancer, the center of treatment should include the family. The health professional must recognize the patient's need for a continuing connection to and support from his or her family at just that time when the family's fears and worries may lead members to withdraw and fail to provide the mutual support and comfort that is so necessary. Our need for our primary-group relationships does not fade once we reach adulthood; the need remains and is implicated in many areas of our lives that fall within the purview of the health professional.

Hospitalism. While much criticism has been leveled at the findings of Spitz regarding what he calls *hospitalism,* his work stands as further testimony to the critical role that early group experiences play in our lives (1945). Spitz observed children in institutions; although they did not lack physical comforts, they lacked the vital social stimulation of other human beings. According to Spitz, these children not only developed lesser intelligence but also were later unresponsive to and disinterested in other persons.

The research of Bowlby, among others, adds further to this picture (1969; 1973). The child who is not provided with a strong mothering relationship tends to have difficulty in forming attachments to other persons. It would seem, then, that one function of our early group experiences is to help us develop intellectually and socially; that is, to help us be capable of later forming those kinds of attachments with others that make the entire fabric of social life and human culture possible. Although he worked with monkeys rather than human children, Harry Harlow (1962) reached a similar conclusion: both parenting and play with peers are essential to adult heterosexual relationships and competency in the tasks of adulthood (e.g., in later being a mother or mothering figure oneself). The peer group forms one of the key primary groups necessary to the development of human beings.

In addition to these effects on the developing child, the reduction of stimulation, including both sensory (e.g., sight, sound, and touch) and social (e.g., interaction and contact with other persons) also has serious consequences for adults. Early research (e.g., Bexton et al., 1954; Scott et al., 1959) has demonstrated a decrement in intellectual functioning and in problem-solving ability when people's normal sensory input is reduced for a period of time. Such people also become more suggestible, open to believing fantastic things (e.g., in ghosts) toward which they otherwise would take a more critical attitude.

Sensory or social isolation, while not usually introduced into adult lives deliberately, nevertheless can result from some medical procedures in which the person is isolated for a period of time—e.g., during radiation therapy.

A similar pattern of *hospitalism* in adults has been described by Sommer and Osmond (1960), among others. It is said to involve such symptoms as the following:

—Deindividuation—a reduced ability to think and act independently; an increased passivity and dependence and loss of a distinct self

—Disculturation—an adoption of institutional attitudes and values and a correspondent loss of earlier attitudes and values

—Isolation and estrangement—a loss of contacts and commitments to things in the outside world

—Stimulus deprivation—a tendency to adapt to a world within the institution, which has a tempo that differs dramatically from that on the outside

These symptoms are said to occur within both patients and staff who must spend a significant amount of time within institutions. The implications of this pattern for both patient care and staff development within institutional settings are clear; use of groups to oppose these symptoms might well become a central aspect of hospital programs.

The Therapeutic Milieu. The concept of the therapeutic community or milieu is a relatively recent one; its origins are primarily in psychiatric settings, but the idea has recently been extended to a consideration of the hospital ward or unit as a therapeutic milieu. Basically, to avoid the effects of hospitalism and sensory limitation, the health professional, especially the person who has greatest hour-by-hour contact with the patient, must attend carefully to creating a total therapeutic context for patient care. The seemingly little attentions and human concerns shown for patients can and do play an important role in recovery. An attitude of extreme clinical detachment, for example, helps contribute to hospitalism and sensory limitation; the patient's milieu, therefore, becomes one that hinders recovery rather than facilitating it. The quality of the milieu is only as good as the people working in it; they must function as a unit. This requires that they deal with some of their own feelings and concerns and with the host of interpersonal issues that develop within any functioning unit. Knowledge and use of group process is essential at two points: (1) in the development and maintenance of a therapeutic atmosphere for the patients; (2) in the functions of the professional staff and their interpersonal issues as they work toward creating a healthful milieu.

We develop into persons by virtue of having contacts with other persons; we remain persons, relatively intact and functioning, as long as such contacts persist. Without our group memberships and belongingness, therefore, we soon experience various symptoms of deficit. Group processes are critical to all human growth and development and to the maintenance of healthful functioning. We return again to this point in a later part of this opening chapter.

The Role of Group Process in Behavior Maintenance and Change

Social psychologist Kurt Lewin formulated the issue of the role of group process in behavior maintenance and change in his analysis of the way in which people change their attitudes and habits (Lewin, 1947a; 1947b; 1958). Although his initial efforts were concerned with changing eating habits by getting persons during wartime to serve less well-known cuts of meat (e.g., kidneys, brains, etc.), the issue remains the same, whether it is eating behavior, smoking behavior, or other health-related attitudes and actions that we need to understand or to change.

Lewin's analysis can be stated in terms of several key ideas:

1. Individual attitudes and habits do not exist in isolation but rather are related to the attitudes and habits of significant groups to which a person belongs or aspires to belong. The teenager, for example, may take up smoking as a habit because a peer group he or she belongs to or would like to join values smoking.

2. We tend to be rewarded with acceptance and a sense of sharing a common view of things when our behavior generally fits within the norms and guidelines of the groups to which we belong. We meet rejection, hostility, or pressure to change when our behavior strays too much from our groups' standards. A nurse working in a setting in which first names only are used is accepted as long as she or he generally follows this policy. Pressure to be like the others is brought to bear if this person breaks the implicit group understanding by using the more formal type of address (Dr. Jones).

3. Lewin suggested that since behaviors are frozen within supportive-group settings, to change those behaviors it is necessary to *unfreeze*

them from their setting. This means that the individual's support on the group in which the behavior is frozen must be reduced or the group's own standards (i.e., norms, guidelines, and implicit or explicit understandings) for the particular behavior must be altered. For example, the smoking teenager's habit may be frozen in a particular group of friends. That behavior can be changed if the teenager's dependence on the group is lessened or if the entire group's evaluation of smoking is changed.

4. To retain the new behavior the person must be within a group context that will support rather than undermine it. This involves a process that Lewin calls *refreezing*—i.e., locating the new behavior in a supportive group, a group whose standards enforce conformity to the new behavior. These ideas of Lewin have obvious relevance to such treatment programs as Alcoholic's Anonymous, to cite one important example. The member of AA both detaches himself from his former "drinking buddies" and simultaneously becomes a member of a group that opposes drinking.

Let us take another example that will help to clarify these points. Suppose that the issue involves helping a person to stop smoking or at minimum to cut down significantly. First, we must recognize that smoking is a habit that not only developed within a group context but is maintained as a habit within a group context. Thus, to change the individual's smoking behavior we must work not only on the person but also on the groups that support that habit. For example, it should be easier to get people to stop smoking if we can bring them and other smokers together in the group to discuss smoking and perhaps collectively agree to reduce it, than by trying to deal with each individual alone. To deal with habits in isolation from the groups to which they are related is not likely to result in change; the person can return to the old ways too easily. Most self-help groups work along these lines. We will examine further facets of group membership and group process in later chapters. For now, however, it is sufficient for us to recognize that so much of what we do and think has not only developed within group settings but is maintained within those settings. Thus to understand or to change poor health habits or to reinforce positive habits, we must work on the level of the membership group(s) rather than on the individual in isolation. And to work on the level of groups requires that we learn group process skills.

It is not stretching the point to suggest that understanding this key function of group process in the change and maintenance of individual attitudes and behaviors is indispensable to our practice. The promotion and maintenance of health means that the health professional must become sensitive to these processes and capable of working with them effectively.

The Role of Group Process in Health Promotion and Maintenance

The preceding discussion emphasized the important functions that groups play in behavior maintenance and change; and this knowledge is critical in the area of health promotion. Let us take an interesting research study from the psychiatric literature to focus more clearly on this point (Cohen et al., 1958).

The problem facing Cohen's psychiatric team involved the treatment of a group of aggressive male and female out-patients through the use of tranquilizing drugs. To provide a proper test of the usefulness of the drugs, a drug group was compared with a matched placebo group over a period of some three months. Measures of the patients' aggressive behavior at home were obtained both before and after drug or placebo treatment. Additional measures were obtained of the patient's home environment. Data from the study are reported in Table 1-1.

The table shows the discrepancies in reported aggressiveness before and after treatment. The negative values indicate that *all* patients showed reductions in their aggressiveness after the three months of treatment. In comparing the data for drug vs. placebo treatment, the most striking finding is that there appears at first to be little apparent difference. A closer examination of the data, however, shows that there is one condition in which the drug produced significantly better results than the placebo; this occurred in the low-conflict family environment. Only when the patient's family setting was low in conflict did the use of a tranquilizing drug prove to be more effective than a placebo. But why?

This research highlights the important function that groups play in health maintenance. The authors suggest several parts to the process. (1) The behavior of those in high-conflict family settings began to

Table 1-1. Average Change in Aggressiveness

	Tranquilizing Drug	Placebo
High-Conflict Family Setting	− 5.67	− 6.50
Low-Conflict Family Setting	− 15.13	− 5.36

change as a function of the drug. (2) These people were in a group in which conflict was the norm, in which aggression and hostility were expected and approved forms of behavior. (3) Any deviation from that normative pattern, as was brought about with the tranquilizing drug, was met with increased pressure to shape up and remain a good group member. (4) In the case of a high-conflict family, being a good group member required being hostile and aggressive. (5) Thus the group process conflicted with the drug treatment program, resulting in an overall ineffectiveness of the drug as compared with the placebo.

Basically, only when the group process reinforces the drug treatment, as in the low-conflict setting, is the treatment program more effective than the placebo. The lesson to be learned is very clear. Anyone involved in the treatment of illness—whether it is psychiatric as in the research example or nonpsychiatric—must carefully know how to evaluate the group factor *and* how to intervene in the group process in the service of health. To ignore the group processes that are involved is to engage in what might prove to be questionable patient care.

As we previously noted, heart disease or cancer cases offer us clear instances in which the medical treatment must be expanded to recognize the group factors that can either support or undermine the program. For example, what is the meaning to the family's existing interaction patterns, or to the business associates, of a change in a person's activity after an MI? The health professional must be aware of the role of group processes in such cases, and must also develop skills in working with relevant processes as part of patient care. Acknowledging group effects is the first step; doing something about them is the next.

The importance of group and social processes in the health continuum cannot be overemphasized. The material that follows provides a convenient summary of some of these important relationships.

The Role of Group and Social Processes in Health Promotion and Maintenance: A Summary Chart

Group and social processes have an important relationship to a number of health factors:

1. *As causative of different states of health*—e.g., the stress of certain kinds of occupations or certain types of roles within groups, such as positions with executive responsibility.

2. *As affecting the reporting of symptoms and disease*—e.g., ethnic

groups vary in their reporting of symptoms (Clausen, 1963; Croog, 1961.)

3. *As affecting the sick role*—e.g., persons and groups vary in their willingness to take on the role of the sick person (e.g., Mechanic & Volkhart, 1960); some evidence suggests the importance of training patients in the role of patient so that they may better participate in their own recovery (Harm & Golden, 1961).

4. *As influencing the course of a disease*—e.g., the effectiveness of medical treatment varies as a function of the patient's role in the family; persons in dependent family roles adapt better to long-term illness at home than persons whose family roles are more active and independent; the latter have more difficulty in home adaptation and seem to benefit more from other care arrangements or from interventions designed to help them adapt better at home (Deutsch, 1960).

5. *In treatment and patient management*—e.g., sensitivity to the group and social factors that may be involved in the patient's maintaining a state of illness is a vital part of the health professional's patient care plan, especially when group process skills are employed in health-producing interventions.

The Role of Group Process in Team Practice

Ours is an era of specialization and often narrow areas of expertise. It is an era of comprehensive health care in which the *team is the key treatment unit* (Steiger, *et al.*, 1960). For most aspects of daily practice, therefore, health professionals find themselves among several others with different kinds of responsibility for managing the care of patients. A person's skills as a team member or organizer are vital to the effectiveness of practice. A team working with heart patients, for example, may consist of the physician, the cardiac nurse, occupational and physical therapists, social service workers, the dietician, and perhaps other specialists as well. Or a team working with colostomy patients may consist of a nurse specialist (helps patients tend to the colostomy so that it will not be a nuisance to them or their families), a nutritionist (helps patients learn about proper foods), a physical therapist (helps patients rebuild strength and recover basic functions), a psychologist or psychiatric nurse (helps patients and families deal with the emotional aspects of the surgery), and perhaps even a patient advocate or social worker (to help deal with the variety of questions and problems that arise in connection with social services). Each person has different functions to carry out, but all share the same concern for the patient's well-being. But as we busy ourselves within our own specialized focus, it is all too easy to forget that the way the team works has serious implications for the patient.

For purposes of illustration, we have chosen an example in which poor or questionable team practice had the potential of producing serious consequences for the patient.

> Dr. Munroe is a second-year resident in family practice at a city hospital. She is just beginning her medical rotation and still sees herself as a student with much to learn. In the context of that hospital, however, she is expected to take on increasing responsibility for her patients. First-year residents turn to her as an expert. Nursing staff, many of whom have much greater expertise than she, nevertheless occupy positions in the hospital's hierarchy that lead them to hesitate to express their judgment, especially when it varies from hers or that of the other doctors. One of Dr. Munroe's patients has developed a severe and disabling back pain. The private physician brings in an orthopedic consultant; both recommend immediate surgical treatment. Though inexperienced and unsure of herself in such matters, Dr. Munroe feels that a more conservative treatment program would be preferable, at least initially. Two of the nurses on the daily rounds share her assessment, but hesitate to support her in the discussions with the private physician and the consultant. They feel it is best to let the medical doctors argue it out on their own. Because she is unsure of her own competencies, Dr. Munroe hesitates to press her view. She makes a few abortive attempts, but these are met with barely disguised hostility and abrasiveness on the part of the private physician: "Who does this resident think she is!" Dr. Munroe senses that to question the doctors too closely is to engage in a battle of egos with them; they would feel threatened and resentful. She decides not to take them on, and lets them decide on the surgery.

This case contains many different illustrative points, not the least of which involves the implications of the power and status relationships between various health professionals for patient care. It shows how a group of persons, all of whom have the care of the patient in mind, and all of whom ostensibly are to function as a team, fail to discuss and evaluate a case openly. The patient's care is given over to the private physician, who has never really been introduced to the good arguments for an alternative treatment program, or to the hour-by-hour assessments of the persons involved in the intimate ongoing care of the patient.

The point is important. We are not arguing that someone other than the physician in charge of the case should be responsible for the patient's overall management. What we are noting is that when team members cannot work effectively together as a unit, the patient does not receive the kind of care that might otherwise be received. We can say that this particular team's group process resulted in what could well be serious consequences for the patient.

The Role of Group Process in Family and Community Work

Except in some rare instances, it is not an exaggeration to suggest that the various states of health are not simply attributes of the individual as such but can be seen to be closely related to the family and the community as well. This is a conclusion consistent with Lewin's position. It is also a position increasingly adopted by health professionals who see illness within a physical/social/psychological framework that is affected by the complex network of group relationships of the patient. The health professional does not simply confront the disease entity that the patient presents, but in addition confronts a person who was, is, and will again be a member of a group network such as a family, a community, etc.

As we have seen, the cancer patient, for example, is much more than a person with a specific set of symptoms. Cancer symptoms are not only individual characteristics with their own history and course of development; they have meaning and consequence for the person's daily living within social groups. If we think of symptoms only as properties of the patient, we lose sight of their broader contexts of meaning. To attend solely to the disease entity as such is to extract it from its group context and thereby to miss what are critical elements in the course and treatment of the disease, as well as the patient's overall health status. Patients typically have many anxieties that include not only physical condition, but extend as well into issues involving the family, the job, the financial situation, etc. There is a need to communicate these anxieties to the health professionals in whose care they are placed (e.g., Brown, 1963).

The less specialized the health professional's role, the greater his or her responsibility for the broad, daily-living aspects of the patient, and the more important are group processes for patient care. In effect the health professional is not confronting a disease, but rather a cast of characters tied together into group networks. Treatment and care therefore require a comprehension of this expanded focus. Although working with families differs in some respects from working with other kinds of groups, there are sufficient similarities in the nature of the group processes that are involved to permit the professional who can learn about groups to make significant headway in family work.

Hospice is the name of a group of some seven nurses, two physicians, and two social workers who worked with thirty-five patients and their families as a unit rather than treating each patient in isolation from his or her family. The patients were all terminally ill but planned to remain at home during their treatment. The health professional staff worked with the families at home to help everyone participate in the patient's care; the terminal illness was considered a matter for family involvement and concern and not just as something happening to the patient or as a matter between the patient and the health professional. The health professionals, in this case, were called upon to be skilled not only in their technical speciality but also in relation to group process as it developed within the families. Their unit of treatment, basically, was the entire family; their skills were therefore required to be broadened to encompass this larger concept of "patient."

Health professionals are often called upon to participate in groups within the community—for example, patient groups, teacher groups, groups formed specifically around particular kinds of health problems (e.g., obesity, sexual dysfunction, cardiac care, etc.). The function of the health professional in such groups may vary, though in the typical case, this person is called on to provide expertise as a consultant; in other instances, the professional may have to be instrumental in organizing the group.

Several noteworthy examples of the use of patient groups as part of health care have recently developed. One program, for example, called the Leukemia Society Outreach Program, is chaired by two health professionals, one of whom is an administrative assistant in pediatric oncology, the other a clinical oncology nurse. The goals of the program can perhaps be best captured through some comments of parents and patients. For example:

My husband and I have never had a chance to sit down and talk with the parents of another child with leukemia. . . . I have never looked another such parent in the eye and I would very much like to.

Through the organization of parents into a group, it is possible to share experiences and provide mutual support; in addition, parents and patients can be provided with information regarding available community services and support facilities.

An adult leukemia patient noted why he needed this type of organization:

> ... there has been one element missing [in my life]. While I had my own thoughts, the love of friends and relatives, and the care of concerned medical staff, I was always aware that I had no other patients to share my thoughts and feelings.

This patient addresses himself to the need for others with a similar illness to come together to discuss their experiences, to universalize what might otherwise appear to be peculiar individualistic feelings, to share problems and possible solutions.

The issue facing the health professional involves the best ways of organizing patient groups or working with groups that are already formed and functioning. Skills in group process and in leadership are clearly essential to effective practice of this sort. These are areas in which definite skills can and must be learned; we are not all intuitively capable of working effectively with groups. Our medical and nursing expertise does not necessarily make us experts as well in group, family, or community work. The health professional cannot simply appear on the scene and practice his or her medical specialty without a like ability to work effectively in and with groups.

The Role of Group Process in Teaching, Training, and Supervision

The practice of health professionals does not only involve them with patients, patient groups, families, or community groups; most are also involved as educators or supervisors, either formally or informally. In formal educational settings, the health professional may organize a small discussion or seminar presentation. Or the health professional may be in a supervisory position in which skills of effective leadership are critical parts of the role. In less formal settings, the professional may be in the role of teacher or supervisor, helping to provide training or supervision to others who are less experienced.

In all cases, the professional must teach, train, or supervise others, individually and in small-group settings. As with any similar endeavor, teaching and supervision do not simply involve transmitting one's own knowledge and skills to another. Rather, an interchange between persons takes place; the effectiveness of the learning depends in great measure on the skills and expertise of the teacher in his or her field of specialization *and* in the knowledge of the group process. Learning to work with a group in training is vital to any health professional who will participate in teaching or supervisory functions. This type of role is especially important in the health professions because so much of the training is based on an in-service or supervisory model.

The Role of Group Process in Organizational Work

Another area within which one's knowledge of group process is important for effective functioning involves organizational structures and informal groups. Most health professionals either center their work in some kind of organizational (i.e., institutional) setting or at various points in their practice must work within the structures and with the informal groups of some organization. Organizations include hospitals, clinics, mental health agencies, educational institutions, and the like. And a significant issue in most institutional settings, but especially hospitals, involves the *coordination* of diverse persons and the effective exercise of authority and leadership. Group process skills are relevant to both of these issues—i.e., the coordination of specialized professionals and the exercise of authority and leadership.

A considerable amount of work in sociology and psychology has demonstrated the important role that small groups play within even the most highly structured and seemingly rigid organization (e.g., Coch & French, 1948; Homans, 1950; Roethlisberger et al., 1939). These tend to be the more informal groups of the sort that Cooley termed primary groups. They criss-cross throughout organizations and provide an often complex network of human relations—one which any practitioner interested in organizational change or effective work within the organization must get to know, understand, and be able to work with.

The health professional may wish to introduce a new practice—for example, a sexuality clinic for patients—and in doing so are likely to run into the problems involved in working within organizations to institute any change. These problems stem not only from the administrative level, but are also rooted in the practices and functioning of the network of informal groups that compose the organization. Many, in fact, see *any* change to be a threat or disturbance to their own status and well-being.

Health professionals may realize that the existing structure of the organization itself thwarts their practice; under such circumstances, the professional must consider ways to change those organizational elements that work to their disadvantage.

> Ms. Robinson, in nurse's training, discovered that the structure of the family planning clinic at which she was interning interfered with her ability to effectively work with her patients. She was expected to provide intake interviews with women coming in for a pelvic examination and for follow-up family planning information and advice. Many of the women were shy and embarrassed about the procedures. They were hesitant to discuss their own needs; they were reluctant to examine the type of family planning they wanted and their feelings about the complex social and psychological issues that were involved. Ms. Robinson sought to help them explore these matters before meeting the physician for the actual examination. She knew that the doctors were busy and took little time to do more than agree to whatever ideas the patient might have. Thus they might recommend an abortion to a young girl who says that is what she would like without ever fully exploring her real feelings on the matter. The clinic itself was located in the hospital's emergency room; thus, the interview rooms that Ms. Robinson used could be taken from her, even during an interview, according to the needs of the E.R. In addition, the doctors were on call upstairs and would often come down for a few quick examinations when their own schedule permitted; this frequently interrupted the intake interview at a very sensitive point. As though this were not enough, doctors frequently had to return to a case upstairs, leaving patients waiting for some time for their return.

This case is illustrative of an organizational arrangement that made Ms. Robinson's work difficult to carry out effectively. Her initial feelings were to blame herself for her poor practice. She lost confidence in her ability to interview and to counsel, and thought several times of leaving nursing entirely—after all, she seemed unable to do her job well. As she came to a better understanding of the organizational structures within which she was carrying out her work, however, she blamed herself less for the problems of practice. At the same time, she was better able to find ways to work more effectively within this arrangement. Her understanding could also have been put to use in attempting to change the clinic's arrangements. Of course, not all organizational features are readily changeable; but there is usually much more flexibility and leeway than may appear initially. A person must be able to develop an understanding of how organizations and groups within organizations work so that his/her own practice can be developed to its fullest potential.

SUMMARY AND CONCLUSIONS

Why does a health professional need to understand group process? The answer to this question is contained in the two words, *scope* and *necessity*. These terms summarize our concern with the role of group process in human growth and health maintenance and in the everyday work of the health practitioner. The scope of the health professional's practice, ranging from direct patient care to working in training and supervisory roles with colleagues and others, makes it apparent that group processes are involved in one way or another at some of the most significant points of practice. It is therefore a necessity for the health professional to develop skill and knowledge concerning group process for effective practice. It is our belief that there are definite, learnable skills involved in group work that can increase the effective practice of the health professional. The purpose of this text is to introduce the learner to those necessary skills.

Table 1–2 summarizes the major points of this chapter, and should be considered as a summarizing guide rather than an exhaustive survey of all users, all target groups, or all functions that are served through knowledge of group process. As the table suggests, however, uses include most persons involved in the health professions. It is obvious that some will find the use of group process more central to their daily practice than others; however, it is our contention, as suggested in this opening chapter, that no one involved in health care can ignore the group processes that are involved in his or her practice. The group side of our human nature is as fundamental as our biological and physical side; it is therefore no mere accident or contemporary fad that the professional team, the family worker, and the group process specialist are becoming increasingly relevant in the health professional's training and practice. Now it is time to get directly to the work of spelling out just what is meant by group process and how to work effectively with groups.

Table 1-2. Group Process for Health Professionals

Users in the Health Professions	Target Groups	Functions
E.g., specialist who must recognize social bases of illness and of treatment	Patient care	For human growth and development

Table 1–2. *(Continued)*

Users in the Health Professions	Target Groups	Functions
E.g., nurse who has responsibility for managing daily living and health care	Patient groups and self-help groups	For health promotion and maintenance
	Other health professionals/team practice	For behavior change and behavior maintenance
E.g., supervisory personnel	Families	
E.g., family practitioners and other primary-care professionals	Community groups	For team organizing, leadership, and management
	Informal groups in institutions	
E.g., teachers and educators	Persons undergoing training and supervision	For patient and family support and education
E.g., public health workers		

Definitions
and Characteristics
of Groups

Most of us realize that people *as individuals* have certain qualities and characteristics. We have an extensive vocabulary of terms in English to describe individuals; one early study suggested that over five percent of the entire lexicon, some 18,000 separate terms, exist to describe traits and qualities that individuals possess (e.g., Allport & Odbert, 1936). We speak of Jim as being *shy* and of Sandra as being *assertive*. These terms describe what we suppose to be the personality traits of Jim and Sandra. What happens when we consider groups of people?

Admittedly, we often use the same terms to refer to the characteristics of a group as we use to describe those of an individual. For example, we describe last Saturday's party as a *rowdy* group; we refer to a football team as *aggesssive*. Yet, we often have difficulty describing characteristics of collectivities and groups. Groups have their own properties and unique characteristics. Individuals who are joined together in a group often act in very different ways: The group may even reveal qualities that no single member in isolation exhibits. This compels us to consider the characteristics that groups possess.

Chapters 2, 3, and 4 direct our understanding to some aspect or characteristic that groups can be said to possess or reveal. Chapter 2 defines the concept of a group. The quality of *interdependence* is central to understanding the ways that groups differ both from individuals alone and collectivities of individuals. Chapter 2 also examines several other qualities that groups possess. We introduce distinctions between types of interdependence (e.g., cooperative vs. competitive), kinds of relationships that characterize different groups (e.g., primary and informal vs. secondary and formal), and the meaning of group membership and group nonmembership.

Chapter 3 introduces the concept of group structure. We argue that a structural analysis, one that seeks to determine the patterns and regularities of a groups' interaction, offers us an important and useful tool. Four types of group structure are examined: roles, communication, attraction, and power.

In Chapter 4 we introduce the implications of two related concepts; group norms and group standards. The concept of a group norm, a rule that guides the interaction of group members, is one characteristic that groups possess that is a critical part of collective behavior.

Unit II offers us a map of the territory of group process. This unit sensitizes us to characteristics and distinctions of which we may have been intuitively aware. They are now systematically laid out to guide our understanding. The chapters in this unit add a storehouse of terms with which we can analyze and understand individual behavior and individual characteristics. This new language is directed toward the analysis, the understanding, and the effective intervention into the world of the group.

2

The Concept of Group and Group Membership

*A*lthough groups are ubiquitous, something that we all participate in all the time, just what are they, really? What characteristics are critical in defining the concept, group? A group refers to associations between two or more persons who are in some kind of *interdependent* relationship to one another. Interdependence is one of the key defining properties of groups as opposed to mere collectivities or aggregates of persons. The concept of interdependence calls our attention to the ways in which persons are *organized* together; it refers to a situation in which what one person does has effects on another person's behavior or perceptions. If people interact and comminicate together, taking one another into account, modifying their own behavior in light of the behavior of others, then we would say that for all practical purposes they belong to a group.

It is helpful to differentiate between a group and a mere aggregate or collectivity of persons who may even share something in common: e.g., all have blue eyes, or all wear white uniforms. Of course, when that shared characteristic becomes relevant to the members' definitions of themselves and others, then we have the beginnings of a *group* . At that moment, people begin to take one another into account, to develop interdependencies and organization. Any shared characteristic could become the basis for group formation: e.g., skin color, sex, clothing, etc. Most of us can recall occasions on which wearing a particular type of clothing has readily identified us and others as members of the "same" group: e.g., as a nurse on the ward rather than as a patient or visitor.

We have said that interdependence is a major defining feature of a group as opposed to a collectivity of persons. Interdependence has two related meanings. First, it focuses on the degree to which persons are organized together so that they no longer act independently, but rather, act interdependently. In this regard, a group is similar to a *system*; it is composed of parts or elements (i.e., the individual members) who function together, who affect and are affected by one another. Second, interdependence refers to the *shared awareness* that persons have of belonging together. While it is possible for persons to be members of a group without awareness of this belongingness, in the usual circumstances, members have a sense of the boundaries of their group; thereby, they have some understanding and awareness about who belongs in and who is out. We return to this point in a later section of this chapter.

A good example of interdependence between two people involves the classic interaction established between Jane and Bob, a not so happily married couple (from Watzlawick et al., 1967). Jane tends to be demanding and to nag Bob; Bob's response to Jane's nagging is to clam up, to withdraw and sit back quietly. This really irks Jane, who then nags Bob even more intensely. In turn, Bob is driven to greater withdrawal. Bob and Jane are members of a small group called a *dyad* or two-person group; it is clearly characterized by its interdependence: Jane's behavior is linked to Bob's and Bob's is linked to Jane's. Each person's response is a function of the other's actions. It would not be stretching the point to say that they are so interdependent that their definition of who each is stands or falls with their mate's response.

INTERDEPENDENCE VS. INDEPENDENCE

As noted, interdependence can be usefully contrasted with independence. Two or more persons are independent when one person's actions have no effect on the others; that is, when they do not form a group or a system. Two small children playing side by side in a sandbox, each wrapped up in a private world of play, could be said to be relatively independent. Jones and Gerard (1967) offer us some examples that sharpen this distinction between independence and the interdependent functioning that describes a group.

Pseudocontingency. Two actors running through a script are only minimally interdependent; each follows the script and uses the other only as a source of cues for his own lines. Jones and Gerard refers to this as *pseudocontingency* because each person's behavior is barely contingent (i.e., influenced by or linked with) the other person's; it is an example of relative independence between the persons.

It is not only script-following actors, however, who engage in such pseudocontingent actions. To the extent that a person plays out a role either rigidly following its plan regardless of the other's responses or totally ignoring the other's responses, he or she may be said to be acting relatively independently. Thus, a true group does not exist. A nurse, for example, who has a technical routine to follow and insists on doing it regardless of the patient's protests, comments, or anxious responses, is acting in a pseudocontingent, relatively independent manner.

Asymmetry. A second relatively independent type of behavior that Jones and Gerard discuss is similar to this last example; they refer to it as *asymmetrically contingent interaction.* In this form, one person's behavior entirely ignores the other's, but the other person's is dependent on the first person's actions—i.e., the other is interdependent with the first. Thus, the nurse may carry out her technical work without any receptivity to the patient; the patient, however, may gauge his or her responses to those of the nurse. Asymmetry is involved in this case in that the nurse's behavior is independent of the patient's, but the patient's is interdependent with the nurse's. Although this type of interaction is not usual in most encounters, in addition to the example cited, it can also occur in various kinds of supervisory and leadership roles. In this case, the leader acts without much regard for the persons being led; they, however, act interdependently with the leader.

Mutuality. Jones and Gerard reserve the term *mutual contingency,* to refer to the more typical form of group interaction. This occurs as each person takes the other's actions into account in setting the course of his or her own actions. Thus there is a mutuality, a true interdependence, and as noted, the essence of a true group.

By now it should be clear that interdependence is not an all-or-none matter—that is, either exists or does not. Rather, it is better understood as a matter of degree. A team of health professionals working together with the common task of planning and providing a patient's health care, for example, is undoubtedly characterized by a much higher degree of interdependence than those same persons sitting in a lecture hall listening to a lecture given by a visiting specialist. Furthermore, as the distinction between types of contingency suggests, members within groups may vary in their own degree of interdependence with the other members of their group. Some may feel themselves more a part of a joint enterprise than others; these latter may experience themselves as fringe members who take little from the others and give little in return. Likewise, some may act with relative independence of the others in their group while others may be mutually contingent (interdependent) with the others.

Summary

Let us briefly summarize. A group may be said to exist whenever two or more persons share some kind of interdependent relationship with one another. This interdependence can be based on different things:

—A common task or purpose that has brought people together (e.g., patient care)

—An attribute shared in common (e.g., in a group in which there are three women and ten men, the women may see their sex as a critical defining characteristic for a subgroup of three within the larger group).

—A pattern of interaction established together (e.g., the nagging wife and the withdrawing husband)

While interdependence involves taking one another into account in the mutual give and take of interaction, adjusting my behavior to yours and vice versa, it is a quality that varies in degree. Some groups are characterized by more interdependence than others; some members are characterized by more interdependence than others.

A NOTE ON GROUP SIZE

Now that we have a definition of the concept of *group*, it will be helpful to examine the issue of group size. For example, we have said that a group exists if it contains *two or more* persons. Is there no lower or upper limit? Does size make a difference?

Surprisingly enough, this is by no means an easy question to answer. We do know that as size increases, so too do the possibilities for relationships among persons. A dyad permits a relationship with only one other; a triad, or three-person group, permits six relationships, the six combinations of the three persons. A group of four allows twenty-five possible relationships. By the time the size of the group reaches seven, there is the possibility for some 966 relationships to develop among the members (Hare, 1962).

Sociologist Georg Simmel (1902–03) developed the fascinating thesis that a distinctly new phenomenon emerges when the size of a group grows from a dyad to a triad. If one person leaves or threatens to leave a dyad, then we no longer have a group. The preservation of the thing known as a group depends on both parties' continued commitment to remain together. Once we get to a triad or to larger formations, however, the life of the group extends beyond that of any one of its members. If one person quits the triad, there nevertheless will remain a two-person group. It is in this sense, therefore, that groups larger than two can be said to have an existence that is more independent of any single member than in the case of a dyad. Simmel also noted that triads permit the formation of coalitions and power relationships of the sort that cannot exist in dyads. Clearly, two members in the triad can join in a coalition to win their position over that of the lone third member.

Others interested in the effects of sheer size have noted a tendency, but only that, for larger groups to produce lower member satisfaction (see Hare, 1962). There is also some indication that beyond a group size of seven, persons have difficulty in observing and evaluating individuals as such; beyond seven, persons tend to relate to others more as members of subgroups or as "those people over there who share the same idea." In other words, with increasing size, persons may relate to one another more as stereotypes or as categories of persons rather than as unique individuals.

Others have noted (e.g., Hare, 1952; 1962) that as the size of a group increases, the time available for members to participate decreases; it becomes more difficult for any one member to speak. In fact, only bolder and more aggressive members may speak as the size of a group increases; those who are generally quiet persons will often be left out of discussions in larger-sized groups. Greater size, however, also permits a greater number and a greater diversity of resources among the group members. With very small groups, composed of only two, three, or even four persons, there is little diversity possible. As size increases, however, the resources potentially available for problem solving increases.

Now, having noted that size apparently makes some difference, at least at the lower and upper limits (e.g., when too many people are present even to discuss matters), we would agree with Cartwright and

Zander (1968), who suggest that the basic group processes involved are highly similar whatever the size, at least within the range of the typical small group: e.g., from two to fifteen persons. Indeed, a dyad may create more pressures on the two members to remain together lest there be no group; yet evidence suggests that similar pressures are brought to bear on members of even larger groups.

One can fruitfully speak of group process without attempting to provide any fine distinction between groups of two through groups of fifteen or so. Within the health professions, groups tend to be relatively small: the dyadic relationship with a patient or a colleague, the team-type relationship, the relationship with the family as a group, the relationship to patient groups or speciality-ward groups, and so forth. The student of group process should remain attentive to the possible effects of group size; however, we are suggesting that within a rather extensive range (e.g., two to fifteen), size may have less effect than other factors.

ANOTHER TYPE OF INTERDEPENDENCE: COOPERATION AND COMPETITION

The defining quality of a group is the interdependence between the members. Interdependence can be relatively low, as in an audience listening to a lecture, or relatively high, as with a surgical team. Also, some group members may be more independent and others more interdependent.

Interdependence, however, differs not only in degree but also in kind. Following the ideas proposed by Morton Deutsch (1953; 1962; 1969) we can distinguish between interdependence based on cooperation and interdependence based on competition. In a *purely* cooperative group, any one member's success or failure signifies success or failure for all the others. For example, if one member of a team does well, then the entire team benefits. By contrast, in a *purely* competitive group, any one member's success signifies failure (or much reduced success) for the others. If one person on the team does well, then none of the others can do well.

These two types describe two extremes of cooperation and competition. In the typical circumstance, these pure types are not encountered. In most groups, a mixture of cooperative and competitive interdependence exists. Thus when the RN does her work well, not only does she benefit, but so too does the patient and the entire team with which she is associated.

It is important to recognize, however, that when we discuss inter-dependence as a critical defining property of a group, we do not thereby mean that groups can only be cooperative. Competitiveness is also a type of interdependence. If you and I are in competition, we must attend to one another's behaviors and adjust our own every bit as much as would be the case were ours a more cooperative situation. However, we would expect different outcomes for a cooperative as compared with a competitive type of interdependence. Research reported by Deutsch has suggested several important differences.

The Benefits of Cooperation

As compared with competition, cooperation results in

—*Greater coordination among members.* This is especially relevant when the group is composed of highly specialized members performing different tasks in which coordination is necessary for effective group performance. If such a group is more competitive than cooperative, individual members seek to do better than others, sacrificing the coordination of the whole group to their own desires to be on top and the best.

—*Greater division of tasks and specialization of functions.* This suggests that cooperation permits persons to specialize more, whereas competition threatens to undo specialization as members try to take on all the tasks for themselves.

—*Greater concern with and attentiveness to other group members.* Interestingly enough, although members of competitive groups are concerned with others' performances, in cooperative groups there is more genuine concern with others: all are in it together and so take more interest in others within their own group.

—*Better understanding of communication among group members.* Communication is rarely an easy matter; all the more important therefore to note that cooperation promotes greater mutual understanding than does competition.

—*Better quality of work.* Although we might have thought that competition within a group helps the quality of work, Deutsch's research suggests this is not the case; competition between different groups might help, but competition internally results in less effective work.

—*Greater sense of "we" and concern for the well-being of the group.* Cooperation promotes a truer sense of belonging to a group with shared goals than does the more splintering effect of competition.

—*Greater friendliness and feelings of self-esteem and esteem for the work of the group.* Cooperation again seems to facilitate individual members' feeling good about themselves and their work; competition may help the winner feel good, but seems to have some negative consequences for the self-esteem of those who do not reach the top.

Implications for Practice

As the listing of outcomes suggests, although competitiveness can be as much a basis for group formation as cooperativeness, a group founded on competitiveness among members who are each vying for the top spot produces negative outcomes to effective teamwork. We will return to this theme at several later points in this text, especially when we examine ways in which leadership can work to increase team effectiveness, in this case, by minimizing internal competitiveness.

What is clearly implied for practice, however, is that there are advantages that evolve from working actively to create a more cooperative than competitive form of interdependence among the members of a group. Cooperation derives from a recognition of shared purposes and shared goals, from a realization of mutual interests rather than divergent interests. While there may be instances in which if I win, you lose, more often than not there is greater room for cooperation than is often realized. Thus individuals must learn to search for their common purposes rather than to emphasize or highlight their differences.

For example, it is not unusual to find team of health specialists divided by issues of status, functioning more competitively than is desirable. The physician competes against the social worker who competes against the nurse; each hopes that his or her practice results in improvement and may even lay claim to having been the one who saved the patient: "It was my work with their family that did it"; "It was my development of a careful diet that did it"; "Without my insightful diagnosis, none of you would even have a patient to work on."

What may sound humorous soon becomes tragic when we realize that each specialist may actually hope that the others fail in their approach and that only one captures the spotlight. Insofar as health promotion and maintenance are truly team-based outcomes, a competitive team can work to thwart the very treatment that may be needed. That is, if the patient's well-being is a function of "the family," "the diet," and "the diagnosis"—as it usually is—then only one specialist who seeks to claim the whole success fails to work in the best interests of the patient.

Cooperation is requisite to teamwork. This demands that each specialist recognizes his or her own part in a larger enterprise; it requires that each search for the common purpose the team shares rather than highlighting individual differences in contribution. This is not simply a Utopian vision, but as we see it, is essential to health care. Practitioners who ignore those skills that facilitate cooperatively based interdependence, therefore, are winning a hollow prize for themselves.

CHARACTERISTICS OF THE SOCIAL RELATIONSHIPS WITHIN GROUPS

Let us return to our discussion, from Chapter 1, of the contribution of Cooley, especially his concept of a primary group; this will provide us with a further analysis of the social relationships within groups. Recall that Cooley introduced the concept of the primary group to refer to the relatively intimate, face-to-face association of persons who felt a strong sense of "we," a sense of camaraderie and of belongingness. This is the type of group relationship that characterizes the family, small friendship groups, and often small, informal groups in work settings. Primary-group relationships are based on close and informal ties that link persons together. The emphasis is on informality and closeness and on the satisfaction of personal needs.

By contrast, we find what can be called secondary or more formal group relationships. These, while often small in size and face to face, are not as intimate and close as primary relationships. Secondary or formal group relationships tend to be those we also encounter at work, when we occupy our work roles and relate to others as nurse to doctor, nurse to nurse, professor to student, health professional to patient. Formal and secondary group ties typically engage only a part of the totality that is us; we are mainly defined by our job and what we do. Secondary-group relationships tend to emphasize work and the accomplishment of some tasks; they emphasize greater rationality and impersonality. Primary or informal group ties encompass more of who we are, extending beyond our work roles and into our personal and often private selves.

All of us belong to both types of groups and experience both kinds of group relationship. Much of the work of health professionals involves the person in more formal, secondary-type groups and relationships. It is the job speciality that has brought persons together with others to form a group or a team. Yet even here more informal, primary-type relationships can and do evolve. Persons form smaller friendship groups within the formal work-group setting.

The student of group process must be sensitive to these different types of group relationships and must develop a facility in working with both. For example, the nurse who is a member of a speciality team is involved in a formal group; yet that same nurse may then work with the patient's family, at which point she is working within a primary group, though not one in which she is a member. Furthermore, that nurse may have her own primary groups in other aspects of her job. Although the basic processes for both types of group relationships are similar, a sensitivity to this distinction can facilitate the work one does. It is usually considered poor practice, for example, to attempt to impose primary-group expectations of personal and more intimate exchange of feelings in a secondary or more formal group; likewise it is usually taken to be peculiar if one seeks to relate more formally within a primary group: e.g., by setting up strict rules of procedure for decision making when primary-type groups tend to rely on more informal, personal bases for reaching their decision.

GROUP FUNCTIONS

The primary–secondary or informal–formal distinction in social relationships has been further refined by other analysts of group processes; they have noted primary-like and secondary-like functions in all groups, whether they be primary or secondary in their dominant form (e.g., Bales, 1955; 1958; 1970; Bion, 1959; Homans, 1950). For example, though a family is a primary group, serving personal needs for its members, it has functions to perform that have a secondary-like quality: e.g., working for a living in order to maintain the family; apportioning family tasks among the members; dealing with budgetary matters. Likewise, though the main concern of a work group (e.g., health professional team) may emphasize impersonality and formal distance between members so that its job can be done, it also must be concerned with the primary-like functions involving member's feelings about one another.

A useful way of focusing on this distinction within all groups is to speak about two types of functions that all groups must serve: task-related or instrumental functions and member-related, interpersonal functions, involving group maintenance. The former are similar to secondary relationships; the latter; to primary relationships. This distinction calls our attention to the two worlds of group process. The one world emphasizes external matters, such as getting the job done or the group's task completed; the other emphasizes internal matters; such as helping to maintain the group's morale and good feelings among the members. Many theorists have employed this same type of distinction:

—Bales speaks about task functions and socioemotional functions

—Homans has referred to a group's external system as contrasted with its internal system

—Bion speaks of a work group as a distinct from an emotionality group

This is an important distinction, one which we will encounter again in several other contexts throughout this text. It informs us that even within highly formalized work groups, based almost entirely on secondary-type relationships (e.g., doctor to nurse; RN to LPN; nurse to patient), primary-type issues are present. While the nurse may be relating to her patient in a rather formal manner, emphasizing her technical expertise, the effectiveness of her work hinges significantly on the patient's acceptance of her care plan. This acceptance depends on the ways in which the nurse has been able to deal with the more primary, informal aspects of her relationship to the patient.

Similarly, a team leader may have substantial expertise and technical know-how in his field and thereby be very skilled in dealing with the external or task functions of the team; yet the team may not function effectively as a team and his own expertise may not be translated into member acceptance because he has failed to deal adequately with internal issues of team maintenance.

The reverse of the preceding is also a realistic possibility. A team leader may emphasize internal matters of group maintenance to the exclusion of external, task-related issues. Thereby, she may have a team in which members have good feelings about one another and in which personal needs for more intimate, close relationships are met, but the team may nevertheless fail in its mission to get its job accomplished. Obviously, therefore, if two sets of function characterize all group processes, both must be adequately handled for effective group functioning. We return to this distinction again in a later section of this chapter.

GROUP MEMBERSHIP: WHO'S IN AND WHO'S OUT?

Who is *in* a group and who is *out*? Who is a member and who is a nonmember? Where does the boundary of the group extend? Who is included within it and who is excluded from it? These are all critical issues of group membership. Membership in some groups, of course, may not appear to be an issue; everyone seems to know who is in and who is out. The more formal the group, the more its boundaries are defined by formal institutions and regulations: e.g., this is a classroom; this is a unit in the hospital. In such settings, the boundary issues may be less troublesome. But even here, membership issues crop up. For example, is the hospital director a member of this group or not? Are the patients on the unit members of the nursing team or not? Are doctors who attend rounds only on occasion members of this group or not? Are persons who hardly participate in the team's work really members or not?

But why is the membership or boundary issue important to understand? Basically, group membership lets us know who we expect to behave like a group member and who we do not expect to behave the way group members should. Being defined as a member of a group places people within the boundary of the system and sets up certain expectations for their behavior toward other members, others' behavior toward them, and members' behavior toward those outside the group. We do not expect nonmembers to act the same way that members are expected to act; we do not bring sanctions to bear on nonmembers for deviating from these expectations; nor do nonmembers expect to be sanctioned (i.e., rewarded or punished) for straying from the behavior expected of members. Therefore, membership indicates who is and who is not included within the power and influence sphere of a group.

Nonmembership

There have been several noteworthy efforts to help define group membership and especially nonmembership (e.g., Merton, 1957; Jackson, 1959). To understand membership and nonmembership, we must know two things: something about the group members and something about the nonmembers. The important element from the perspective of the group members involves what Jackson has termed *acceptance* and Merton, *eligibility*.

Eligibility.   Acceptance or eligibility refers to the degree to which there exists a position in the group for a nonmember. We can speak of a dimension of eligibility. At one end, we have nonmembers who are defined as eligible for membership; for them acceptance is a real possibility. At the other end, we have nonmembers who are ineligible for membership, for whom negative acceptance (rejection) is the real possibility.

For example, nursing has specific degree requirements for its membership; persons who have the degree are eligible for membership in numerous groups within nursing, whereas persons without the proper degree are ineligible, at least until they obtain their degree. Until that time, they are excluded from membership. A group that actively excludes persons because of their age, their sex, their race, their religion, or similar characteristics is one that declares many types of persons to be ineligible for membership. Caste systems in India provide one such example, as do many kinds of professional and private associations in the United States. The family typically defines as ineligible for membership all those persons not linked by blood or by marriage into the group. If marriage across religious lines, for example, is not acceptable to a given family, then its boundaries extend to include as potential members only those of the same religion as existing family members. Intermarriage thereby fails to extend the group's boundaries; rather, both the blood kin and that person's spouse are rejected.

Attraction.   The second element in our equation for understanding the issues of membership and nonmembership is derived from the nonmembers themselves. Jackson refers to this dimension as *attraction*, while for Merton it involves the nonmembers' *attitudes toward becoming a member*. Again, we have a dimension. One end represents positive attraction; the nonmember aspires to belong to the group. At the other end, we have negative attraction; the nonmember is actively motivated not to belong to the group.

When we apply the concept of attraction to actual group members rather than to nonmembers, we are dealing with the very important concept of *group cohesiveness*. Cohesiveness is based on an analysis of a groups' total profile with respect to members' attraction to the group. A group is said to be highly cohesive and thereby likely to function effectively insofar as all persons who are members are highly attracted to their group; low cohesiveness represents a condition in which members generally belong to the group but are not highly attracted to this membership. When we are dealing with nonmembers, however, the issue is not one of cohesiveness, but rather involves the nonmembers' attitudes toward becoming a member.

Table 2–1 provides a summary of *nonmember types* based on an analysis of the group's definition of a person's eligibility for membership and the nonmember's attraction toward joining the group. A plus (+) indicates positive eligibility or a positive attitude toward joining; a minus (−) indicates ineligibility or negative attraction.

Table 2–1 tells us several important things. The analysis suggests that nonmembership is a highly differentiated matter. The *in* vs. *out* issue, therefore, is more complex than we might otherwise have thought. There are various ways of being outside the boundaries of a group. But, even more significantly, these different ways of being outside have different implications for those who are inside: i.e., for the members. Antagonistic nonmembers may force a group toward internal cohesiveness almost as a defense against the hostility from outside. On the other hand, marginality is undoubtedly more painful for the nonmember than for the members; it describes a nonmember who would like to be a member but who is not eligible for such membership. Of course, it may have some appeal to a group because it can enable the members to feel very exclusive.

Marginality

The student of group process can benefit substantially from a knowledge of these types of nonmembers. For example, a marginal nonmember, as we have noted, is in an especially difficult, often disturbing position vis-à-vis a particular group. Marginal people crave acceptance but are not yet eligible and so really do not know where they stand in relation to others. This could describe the student nurse who

Table 2-1. Types of Nonmembers

	Eligibility	Attraction to Join
Candidate for membership	+	+
Autonomous nonmember	+	−
Marginal nonmember	−	+
Antagonistic nonmember	−	−

is doing an internship at a hospital and is not yet fully accepted as a member of the professional staff. She is marginal and will typically reflect some of the symptoms of this marginality: e.g., high anxiety levels, confusion, excessive efforts to please or excessive rebellion, loneliness, anger, perhaps despair and depression. Knowing that a person is marginal to a group can not only help our diagnosis of some of that person's difficulties; it can also facilitate our intervention on his or her behalf. If we are the leader or organizer of the group, we can actively invite the marginal person in; even though the person is not, strictly speaking, eligible for full membership, he or she can be brought in and treated more as a member and less as a marginal person.

Groups we may deal with in practice (e.g., families and patient groups) may also have marginal nonmembers. It is not that unusual to find adolescents, for example, to be marginal within their own families. Technically they belong but psychologically they are not yet considered eligible for full adult status within the family. They are marginal and show many of the symptoms of their marginality. Again, the health, professional working with this group can help undo the adolescents' marginality: e.g., working to include the adolescent in the family, helping the family explore the issue of marginality, and so forth.

The Candidate and the Autonomous Nonmember

Two further interesting cases of nonmembership involve those who are candidates and those who are autonomous.

A group that confronts many autonomous nonmembers—that is, those who are eligible for membership but who are not attracted to membership—finds itself in a difficult position. What must it mean for members to know that many eligibles do not wish to join? For example, what would the ANA or AMA be like if few of those eligible for membership actually became members? As Merton noted, "Rejection by eligibles symbolizes the relative weakness of the group by emphasizing its incompleteness of membership just as it symbolizes the relative dubiety of its norms and values which are not accepted by those to whom they should in principle apply" (1957, p. 291).

For example, a residency program in Family Practice gauges its own value by computing a matching score based on comparing the number of high-ranking applicants it accepts with the number who actually accept membership in the program. A high percentage indicates that the program is able to match well—that is, to attract those persons to join the group that it most wants to join. A low percentage, by contrast, signifies a basic weakness in the group; few of those it wants to join seek to join it; they go elsewhere. The morale of the members of the program is significantly affected by these percentages. The low-percentage match indicates, as Merton has noted, that something about the group's norms, values, and effectiveness is doubtful. Or, take another example.

> Teaching Team A at a school of nursing has a longstanding reputation as being high in conflict, a difficult group to work with. Each year the team must search for new members to complete its speciality teaching requirements. Many candidates are eligible to join the team; the faculty is large and there are additional openings for several new persons to be hired. However, literally none of those many who are eligible wants to join the team. Team A can be contrasted with Team B at the same school; all of the eligible candidates are eager to join Team B. Its reputation is of a better, more harmonious work group, one in which the person can function more effectively as a nurse-educator.

In terms of Table 2–1, Team A has many autonomous nonmembers, while Team B has many candidates for membership. The presence of so many autonomous nonmembers lowers the morale and potential effectiveness of Team A; the existence of many candidates, on the other hand, boosts the morale and effectiveness of Team B.

The importance of group morale for group effectiveness is rather apparent. What may not be as apparent, however, is the implication of this analysis of nonmembership for understanding one of the bases for high or low morale. The student of group process will benefit substantially from a recognition that *morale is affected by nonmembers as well as by members.* Diagnosing a morale issue, therefore, may require an understanding of who does *not* belong to the group. It is difficult for a group to maintain itself or to think well of itself if too many eligible members fail to join. The group's leader might do well to consider the implication of these nonmembers for group functioning.

REFERENCE GROUPS AND MEMBERSHIP GROUPS

The concept of a nonmember who is a candidate for membership, the person who is both positively attracted to membership in the group and is eligible for membership, introduces us to the important idea of *reference group* (see Hyman, 1942; Newcomb, 1943; 1958). When we speak of a reference group, we mean a group in which a person either may or may not have membership; in either case, it is a group the person uses as a reference source for his or her own attitudes, values, and behaviors.

There are three possibilities. First, a reference group may also be a membership group. This is a group the person belongs to, identifies with, and uses to guide his or her own points of view. Jackson refers to this as *psychological membership* in a group. Second, a person may be a member of a group, yet not consider it to be his or her reference group. Jackson refers to this person as a *rebellious member*. Although such people belong to the group, they are negatively attracted to it; they use other groups as the source of their own values and attitudes. For example, a person may be a member of a team and yet so dislike membership on that team that he adopts the values of another team as his own rather than his own team's values.

Finally, a person may not be a member of the group and yet be a candidate for membership; this person uses the group she is not yet in as a basis for her own attitudes, values, and behaviors. The process, termed *anticipatory socialization*, usually occurs under these circumstances. The nonmember candidate begins to act in the way that actual members act, adopting the members' mannerisms, clothing (if possible), values, and such. This is anticipatory socialization in that it helps prepare the candidate prior to membership for taking on the characteristics proper to actual membership. Thus, the person, anticipating membership, begins to become socialized into the ways of membership.

Nursing students in training will be eligible for membership in many groups in their field; their training may be seen as involving anticipatory socialization, by which process they begin to adopt the perspectives of those groups for which they are candidates for membership though not yet actual members. In this way, when they graduate and become actual members, they are already able to behave as members do.

The reference-group concept has proved very useful for understanding a variety of phenomena about human behavior. In addition to examining the effects of actual group membership on member behavior, the reference-group concept informs us that groups influence nonmembers who aspire to belong and are candidates for membership. Therefore, in understanding group process, we must expand our focus and examine both membership groups and nonmembership, reference groups.

The reference-group concept also helps us understand how persons resist being influenced or affected by their present membership groups. A student, for example, may reject her university as a reference group even though it is her membership group. She may successfully accomplish this by maintaining her family as her key reference group, retaining its attitudes and values rather than adopting, for example, the more liberal attitudes of her university membership group (e.g., Newcomb, 1958).

MEMBERSHIP ALTERNATIVES AND MEMBERSHIP TYPES

Thibaut and Kelley (1959) provide us with two further concepts that amplify our understanding of the process involved in group membership. We examine additional aspects of their theory in Chapter 7. These investigators make a distinction between a group member's *attraction* to the group and his or her *dependency* on the group. As we have discussed, a member's attraction refers to the degree to which that person likes or dislikes being in the group. Dependency, however, is a somewhat different dimension of membership. To be dependent on a group means not to have equally attractive alternative groups for membership. A member might be highly dependent on one particular group because there are no other groups that are more attractive or because the costs involved in leaving the group reduce the attractiveness of other possible alternatives.

For example, an RN may have to retain her employment in a given hospital in a community for family reasons. In a tight job market, she may have few alternative employment possibilities (i.e., few alternative group memberships) and so is highly dependent on her present group membership. Likewise, the costs involved in moving out of the community to find work and memberships elsewhere may be so great as to make any alternatives less attractive. By contrast, in a good job market or with a different family situation, mobility possibilities may be so great that dependency on any one group may be low; numerous alternatives help the RN feel relatively independent of any one membership.

A member's dependency on a group is a matter of degree; it can have important implications for how that member functions within the group and how the group as a whole functions. A member who feels minimally dependent on a group, having many equally attractive alternatives, for example, will be less influenced by the group than will a person who is more highly dependent; the latter is likely to go along with the group because no other choices are available. Obviously, resistance to group influence can be greater if people can simply pack up and leave than if that is the only group in town and they must stay. High dependence, of course, does not necessarily make for an effective work group; just the opposite possibility also exists. The burning resentment of those who have few alternatives often shows up in poor work performance, lateness, refusal to take responsibility for tasks that must be done, general apathy, nonparticipation, and so forth.

In the Thibaut and Kelley analysis, attraction and dependency can vary. Four possibilities can be represented:

	Attraction	*Dependency*
Type A	High	High
Type B	High	Low
Type C	Low	High
Type D	Low	Low

Type A describes the member who is attracted to the group and highly dependent on it; we would not expect great resistance or resentment in such a member. Although such people have few alternatives to their present group membership, they are highly satisfied with the situation. Type B describes people who are highly attracted to the group but not dependent on it; these members have alternatives and so are more able to resist undue group pressure; yet they need not resent this group, to which they are highly attracted. Type C describes people who are more highly dependent on the group than attracted to it. These are types of members who harbor much resentment; they are literally stuck in a setting that is not much to their liking. Type D describes what might best be termed apathetic group members who are neither very attracted to the group nor highly dependent on it; alternatives do exist, but they seem to remain in the group, showing neither enthusiasm nor resistance.

SUMMARY AND CONCLUSIONS

This chapter has sought to answer two related questions: What is a group? and What does group membership mean? The essential definition of *group* involves the idea of interdependence: persons are interdependent insofar as they take one another into consideration in determining their own behavior; what each does has effects on the other and vice versa. We noted that interdependence is a matter of degree and a matter of kind. There is a range of interdependence, from little or none (none would be true independence in which one's behavior is not affected by anothers), through a middle range (e.g., members of an audience), to relatively high (e.g., members of a group in which each person acts in consideration of the actions of the others). In terms of types, interdependence can involve cooperation or competition. We noted how a cooperatively based interdependence seems generally more effective than one based on competition. We next examined different types of social relationships within groups, noting the important difference between formal relations and task functions on the one hand and informal relations and socioemotional functions on the other. We concluded the chapter with a consideration of the complex meaning of group membership, noting how different types of nonmembership produce different consequences for the group as well as for the nonmember.

IMPLICATIONS FOR PRACTICE

We called attention at several points throughout this chapter to some of the implications of this analysis of group and group membership for the practitioner of group process. Basically and briefly, the concepts introduced in this chapter are designed to sensitize the health professional to the complex set of issues and meanings of group membership and of interdependence. These ideas are essential for anyone who must diagnose and intervene in issues involving group work and teamwork, whether these be focused on peer and colleague groups, on family and patient groups, or on community and organizational groups. Diagnoses and intervention in issues of group morale and individual marginality are especially dependent on knowledge of the concepts introduced in this chapter.

Likewise, by introducing a more complex picture of group membership, we have implied that nonmembers of groups can be and often are as significant to our understanding of group process as actual, physically present members. Nonmembers who are autonomous (eligible but refuse to join) can threaten the integrity of the group itself. In addition, a membership or a nonmembership reference group can be an important locus for an individual's values and behaviors. To ignore a person's reference groups in addition to groups of his or her actual, ongoing membership is to fail to fully grasp the forces that have an impact on that individual's life and well-being.

The practitioner of group process, therefore, must learn to become sensitive to a concept of group and group process that has very extensive and typically psychological rather than purely physical boundaries. That is, the boundaries of a group and hence the effects of a group are not simply represented by the persons who are now present and gathered; boundaries can include persons who are psychologically present as reference points for the individual's attitudes, values, and behaviors. These psychological groups form an important part of our understanding of group process effects.

3

Structural Characteristics
of Groups

THE CONCEPT OF STRUCTURE

No understanding of groups is complete without an examination of the concept of *group structure*. Few human relationships are without structure. When we refer to the structure of a relationship or the structure of a group, we focus on the ways in which persons are involved in (a) ordered arrangements (b) that define and regulate their behavior and (c) that provide a patterned constancy and stability to their behavior together (Nadel, 1957).

Ordered Arrangements. In focusing on structure, we attempt to uncover the recurring patterns of relationship and interaction that exist without necessarily specifying who the persons are that participate in these ordered arrangements. There can be a total shift of personnel—old members leave and new members enter—yet the structural constraints on behavior remain the same. In music, for example, it is possible to speak about the structure of a symphony or the structure of a sonata without specifying the exact notes and melodies that are involved. Structure describes an arrangement of the parts (e.g., musical notes, group members, etc.) that is maintained regardless of what specific parts are involved. For example, in an organization that is described as having a *tall* rather than a *flat* structure of authority and decisionmaking, persons on top make decisions that are handed down to those below (e.g., Porter & Lawler, 1964). The flat structure is more egalitarian; decisionmaking is shared among all persons rather than being handed down from the top. The terms "tall" and "flat" describe the power structure of the organization; regardless of what specific individuals are involved within it, they are constrained by the nature of the structure to behave in particular ways.

Constraints. The second part of this three-part definition of group structure calls attention to this defining and regulating (i.e., constraining) quality. If a composer were to write a sonata, for example, he or she would be constrained to use the structural arrangements that define the composition as a sonata regardless of the particular notes that were used. In a similar manner, the structure of a group defines and regulates the behavior of the persons involved in it. Persons high up in a tall organization are expected to exercise authority and hand down decisions just as those in a flat structure are expected to share more equally in decisionmaking.

To take another example, the role structure of the society and its organizations (e.g., a hospital) defines a nurse's role and a doctor's role. To be sure, there may be variations in these definitions; certain aspects of the roles are more rigidly defined than other aspects. Nevertheless, a role description is a structural analysis. It informs us that regardless of which actual doctors and nurses are involved, they will be constrained by their roles to act in particular ways toward each other and toward their patients.

Knowing this structural feature of the relationship of the roles of nurse and doctor allows us to make some reasonable assessments of the behavior to expect even before we know which particular nurse and which particular doctor will actually be working together. Roles, however, compose only one of several structural features; we will shortly examine roles as well as the other important structural characteristics of groups. In all cases, however, the point remains: structures are institutionally defined arrangements that regulate and constrain the behavior of whatever specific persons are involved working in them.

Stability. The third aspect of the definition of group structure informs us that structures provide a patterned constancy and stability to the behavior of the persons involved in the structure. Recall that structural properties of a group are defined independently of the particular persons who are members of the group; a change in membership thus need not produce a change in group structure. Constancy and stability are provided by the structural pattern rather than by any necessary constancy of personnel. A sonata is a sonata regardless of who has composed it, who performs it, and what notes are used in it. The constancy that permits us to recognize it as a sonata exists in and is carried by its musical structure.

It may be disconcerting to think in these terms. Nevertheless, it is important for the student of group process to understand that much that is constant and stable about group and individual behavior within groups is carried by the constancy of group structure rather than by a constancy of personnel. In very practical terms, this means that the personnel can be changed, many different personalities can be involved, and yet the group as such remains relatively constant and stable. A hospital is structurally similar and constant over time even when its personnel rotates out and even when the personalities of the specific individuals involved varies.

Structural Analysis

It is important to analyze people's behavior in terms of the group structures they are in as well as in terms of individual personal qualities. This is a crucial point. Too often, we attribute behavior to something about personality, failing thereby to locate its cause within the structure (e.g., the role) of the group or organization. For example, a certain health professional may behave in an autocratic manner; she acts impersonally and unilaterally; she gives direction to others and seems to ignore or discount her subordinates' feelings and ideas. Do we attribute this behavior to something about this individual's personality? Do we say, "She is just a bossy dictator, a power-hungry professional"? Or are we also sensitive to the structural constraints that influence that person's behavior? Do we see her behavior as shaped by her position within a hospital organization, for example? To make a structural analysis of behavior is to search for those arrangements within the system (e.g., group or organization) that constrain the person's behavior rather than searching for something deep within his or her personality.

In Chapter 1, in the discussion of hospitalism as it affects both patients and staff, we introduced a structural analysis of behavior. The constraints of a particular kind of hospital or unit structure, one in which staff members perform routine duties in a distant and formal way—technically proficient but humanly sterile—give rise to a behavioral syndrome called hospitalism. Our search for the bases of this syndrome must focus on the structural patterns within the organization that promote this behavior rather than on qualities within the personalities of either the patients or the staff. In many respects, even the most humane and concerned health professional who is placed within this type of organizational structure will in time come to take on many of the behavioral attributes of "hospitalism." Knowledge of group structure is thereby vital to the health professional who would both diagnose a group's problems and know something about the proper intervention strategy to employ.

Of course, there are limits to these constraints. A change in personnel, a unique coalescence of different personalities, can and does have consequences for the existing structure of a group or organization such as a hospital. New structures emerge as old structures are changed. In general, however, many of the constancies and the stabilities of behavior are carried by structures. Thus, even as the old structure gives way to the new—as persons bring new ways of interacting or as tasks demand different structures for their accomplishment—the new establishes its own ordered arrangements of the individuals who are working together.

It will be helpful at this point to examine several of the major types of group structure that are typically encountered; these help define some of the important characteristics of groups as seen from a structural perspective. We will focus on the following four: roles, communication, attraction, and power.

ROLE STRUCTURES

Of all the types of group structure, role structures are perhaps the most familiar and most easily understood (see Biddle & Thomas, 1966; Sarbin & Allen, 1968). This should come as no surprise. The concept of role is not used solely by sociologists or psychologists—it is a common term of analysis used by persons in their everyday dealings with one another. All societies, all groups, and all persons differentiate and classify populations into roles—that is, into positions that individuals take on and that carry with them certain expected behaviors and responsibilities (doctor, nurse, patient, teacher, director, mother, old man, woman, child, etc.).

Ascribed vs. Achieved Roles

Social scientists have found it useful to distinguish between two ways in which roles are classified (e.g., Linton, 1936). The first is termed *ascriptive*. *Ascribed roles* are based on certain characteristics that are intrinsic to the persons involved: e.g., male, female, young, old. The second involves *achievement*. *Achieved roles* are those that persons accomplish or achieve by virtue of their activities, things they do well, particular interests and abilities they have: e.g., doctor, nurse, president, etc. Not every instance of role behavior can be neatly classified as being either ascribed or achieved. The central emphasis, however, is clear. Ascribed roles are a function of some qualities that persons have that are generally beyond their control, such as their sex and their age. Achieved roles are a function of qualities over which they tend to have greater control, such as their occupation.

As with all structural characteristics, roles define and regulate the behavior of those who occupy them. Behavior is regulated by both our ascribed and our achieved roles. Sex and age, for example are ascribed characteristics that carry with them certain expectations for proper behavior; likewise, achieved roles define and constrain persons to certain proper behavior.

Fit Between Role and Self

Some roles fit certain people better than others. When there is a lack of fit between what the role demands and what the person feels capable of doing, we usually note symptoms of tension and discomfort both for the individual and for the particular role system (e.g., the group) in which the person is involved. For example, a supervisory position entails a role with expectations for the behavior of whoever occupies that position. If Adams is made supervisor, and acts in a withdrawn manner, hesitating to take the initiative to provide leadership and supervision, two consequences may follow. First, she may experience discomfort as she tries to behave in ways that fit the role's requirements but which do not fit her own personal ways of behaving. In time, she may grow into the role and become more the type of person it demands; or she may forever be at war with it. Second, the group may suffer when Adams does not enact her role properly. The role structure of a group usually consists of an interlocking network of several roles; when one or more does not function, the others in the network likewise have difficulty. The supervisor who does not take on the responsibilities proper to that role thereby leaves a gaping hole in the group's role structure.

Once again, a structural analysis (a role analysis, in this case) would be helpful both for understanding and intervening in a difficult group situation. The supervisor in our example has a job that is ill-suited to her character. This creates problems for her and for her group. The source of the problem, however, is structural in that it involves the particular role constraints that conflict with Adams' personality. Several options for change are now apparent. For example, Adams can delegate greater leadership responsibility to others; or she can try to work in a more egalitarian manner with the group. In this way, the group structure is changed from tall to flat and thereby the supervisory role is transformed from one requiring greater dominance to one requiring a more democratic arrangement. Thus we see that a recognition of the structural basis of a problem can help in bringing about a structural solution.

Conflict Between Different Roles

All of us occupy more than one role; we may be mother or father and doctor; we may be teacher by day and student by night. We can usually avoid the difficulties involved in having to enact both roles simultaneously by segregating them in time or in place. For example, we can be parent at home and nurse at work; we do our parenting at one time and fulfill our obligations as nurse at another time. There are moments, however, when a conflict develops between the several roles we occupy. This conflict may occur, for example, when the same job is defined differently for us by the different persons with whom we interact; that is, our role means one thing to one person and something different to another. We are placed in a conflict, then, between these differing conceptions of our role. In a sense, it is a conflict between two sets of roles.

The classic example of this conflict occurs for people who occupy middle-level positions within an organization (e.g., Stouffer et al., 1949a, b). Those who are superior to them in the organization's hierarchy define their role in one way, usually seeing them as representative of the administrative hierarchy; those who are below them in the organization define their role in a very different way, usually seeing them as a friend, one of their own group. There is little chance for people caught in the middle to segregate their roles by time or place; they are both, at the same time and in the same place.

One version of this conflict between two roles is highlighted by the following example:

A nursing supervisor enrolled for a course in interviewing and counseling techniques, hoping to learn how to better deal with what she felt to be a difficult situation. As supervisor, she was expected to be a rather stern, authoritative person, making certain that the young nurses under her supervision got their work done properly. Yet she was also expected to provide these younger and less experienced nurses with a warm and supportive figure to whom they could turn in their own moments of need and personal crisis. The nursing supervisor complained that she just didn't know how to take on both of these conflicting roles at the same time. How could she be both stern/authoritative and warm/supportive?

As was noted earlier, roles are so interlocked that a problem for the role occupant becomes a problem for everyone tied into that same role relationship. In the case of the nursing supervisor, not only did she face a problem, but so too did all the nurses she was supervising. Who was she from their perspective? Let us suppose that they had problems and wanted to seek some support from her. When they approached her, how could they know which role she was enacting? Was she the stern figure who would reject their claims for support as she tried to get them to do their work more efficiently? Or was she the warm figure to whom they could turn for a shoulder to cry on and support for their confusion? Her problem, in other words, was their problem as well.

It is reasonable to refer to the kinds of conflict expressed in the previous example as *structural*. Any person who occupies roles of the sort described would experience conflict. The conflict is built into the structure of the group or organization; in this regard, therefore, it is not like the conflict between self and role. The latter entails conflict for only certain kinds of persons. To recognize something as involving a structural conflict rather than a more personal one can often alleviate some of the strains that people feel. Rather than always putting the blame on themselves, they can see the structural context within which the conflict is generated. To be sure, the pain and anguish will not thereby be magically dissipated, but seeing its origin in structural terms can help considerably.

Understanding the nature of conflict in structural rather than in personal terms can also provide a clue as to its resolution. A structural conflict will not fade simply with psychotherapy or a happy attitude toward one's work; such conflicts require a solution that attacks the proper level of the problem: that is, a structural solution is required. Organizational changes are required to alleviate the personal problems that derive from these kinds of structural arrangements. On the other hand, where the organization remains resistant to change or where the efforts involved in seeking to affect such change seem beyond one's abilities, the best tactic may be to bite the bullet and bear the structural conflict or get out. Because few conflicts are purely personal or purely structural, a compromise between changing one's own outlook somewhat and seeking to somewhat modify the organizational structure may work best in the long run.

Group Roles

Analysts of group process have noted role structures in all groups, including both formal groups that emphasize task functions and informal groups that emphasize more social functions. Role structures in groups often overlap with the prevailing communication and power structures. For example, the differentiation between group leader and members describes a feature of both the group's role structure and its power structure. Similarly, an analysis of members into roles based on their predominant mode of communicating and interacting proves informative about both the role structure and the communication structure of the group. Research reported by Bales has suggested two major roles within all groups based on the types of communication that describe the particular role (1958). He refers to these as *task roles* and socioemotional or *maintenance roles.*

Task and Social Specialists. Bales' analysis argues that all groups must develop role structures in order to deal with two kinds of problems: the external problem of successfully coping with the task they have undertaken; and the internal problem of successfully dealing with inter-member relations. Speciality roles tend to emerge within groups to handle each type of problem. A *task specialist* has to do with a role or set of roles that emphasize getting the job done, working in ways that are more efficient for dealing with the group's tasks. A *social specialist* involves a role or set of roles that emphasize keeping the group working together in relative harmony, dealing with conflicts with the group, and generally helping with issues of group maintenance.

Based on their own and others' observations of many groups, Benne and Sheats (1948) expanded somewhat on Bales' analysis. They not only described further types of roles within the task and the group maintenance areas, but in addition they introduced a third set of roles involving what they termed *individual functions*. This third category includes roles that serve individual members' own personal needs rather than those of the group as a whole. Table 3–1 summarizes several examples of their role analysis.

As with Bales' analysis, the roles proposed by Benne and Sheats suggest an aspect of group structure in which any number of group members may participate. Dr. Winslow, for example, may take on the individualistic role of dominator in one session and take on the task role of initiator in another. Nurse Coopersmith might serve the task function of coordinator in one session or one part of a group meeting and take on the maintenance role of harmonizer in another part of

Table 3-1. Member Roles Within Groups

ROLES INVOLVING TASK FUNCTIONS

Initiator: involves proposing new ideas, new directions, new tasks, new methods.

Elaborator: involves expanding on existing suggestions, developing further meanings to the group's plans.

Evaluator: involves critically evaluating ideas, proposals, and plans, examining the practicality of proposals, the effectiveness of procedures.

Coordinator: involves helping to pull ideas and themes together, to clarify suggestions that have been made, to help various subgroups work more effectively together toward their common goals.

ROLES INVOLVING GROUP MAINTENANCE FUNCTIONS

Encourager: involves offering praise and agreement with other members; involves communicating acceptance of others and their ideas and an openness to differences within the group.

Harmonizer: involves mediating conflicts and disagreements that crop up, trying to relieve or reduce tension within the group.

Compromiser: involves seeking a position between contending sides, seeking a compromise that all parties can accept.

ROLES INVOLVING PRIMARILY PERSONAL, INDIVIDUALISTIC FUNCTIONS

Aggressor: involves acting negatively, with hostility toward other members, denigrating others' contributions, attacking the group and its members.

Recognition-Seeker: involves efforts to call attention to one's own activities, to boast, to redirect things toward oneself.

Help-seeker or confessor: involves using the group as a vehicle either to gain sympathy or to accomplish personal insights and personal satisfactions without consideration for others or the group as a whole.

Dominator: involves asserting authority and seeking to manipulate others so as to be in control of everything that happens.

---

that same meeting or in another session. These describe patterned ways of behaving within groups and not necessarily particular people. Naturally, a given individual may characteristically adopt one kind of role or another. Thus, Nurse Coopersmith may typically take on a mixture of task and maintenance functions, while Dr. Winslow typically functions within the individualistic area.

What is important to understand about Bales' analysis and that of Benne and Sheats is that role structures emerge within a group in order to serve certain basic functions that are necessary for the group's success. Some functions are concerned with getting the external task completed, while other functions are concerned with maintaining the group while it works together. Both sets of functions must be served for the group to be effective. Individualistic roles do not serve these necessary group functions, but rather serve member's personal needs often at the expense of the group.

When Bales speaks of a role specialist such as a task specialist, he is referring to a set of communicative behaviors that attend to task functions. These behaviors involve some of the specific activities that Benne and Sheats list under their category: e.g., initiating, elaborating, evaluating, coordinating. While these two sets of functions, task and maintenance, must be served and roles must emerge to deal with them, the particular individuals who come forward to serve them can vary. As with all aspects of group structure, the specific personnel may change within a group, but these two functions and the roles that serve them remain.

The Gatekeeper.   Lewin's analysis (1958) of the use of group processes in behavior maintenance and change (recall Chapter 1) introduces us to another role within groups: that of *gatekeeper*. It was Lewin's suggestion that a key role within any group is the one that provides an entry point from the outside into the group. In the examples he studied, involving changing the eating habits of families, he suggested that the wife was the gatekeeper to the family's dinner table. That is, she was in the key position to determine what food was actually served. Thus, to affect a change in the gatekeeper would be to affect a change in the entire family's eating habits.

The student of group process, especially in the health professions, must be sensitive to this type of group role. To find the gatekeeper of a group is to find the key role that permits the outsider (e.g., the health professional) entry into the group. As in Lewin's own example, in many families, the health care issues are focused around the wife and mother as the gatekeeper. It is she, therefore, who occupies the critical position within the family when it comes to making health-related decisions. This may not be true in all families; but identifying the gatekeeper is critical for anyone who needs to work with that group.

In many instances, group leaders may need to know who is the gatekeeper to an informal clique or subgroup within their own larger group in order to have effective access to all members of the group. For example, a health professional team may consist of eight persons, three of whom could be said to form a subgroup of close friends within the larger group of eight. To work most effectively with the entire group, the team's leader would benefit from knowing who was the gatekeeper to that three-person subgroup. To reach that gatekeeper and influence his or her behavior would be the most effective way to reach all members of the subgroup. Indeed, as we can recall from Lewin's analysis in Chapter 1, trying to influence a member of that subgroup without due consideration for the dynamics of the subgroup, especially its organization around the gatekeeper, might prove to be a wasted effort.

As in the other cases we have been considering, a structural role analysis proves to be an essential first step in planning and carrying out intervention into a group. Much time and effort are wasted by a health professional, for example, who makes contact with a family through one of the less influential members rather than the gatekeeper. It may be possible to convince that person of the need for a change in the family's health practices, but this may not be effective in producing a change for the entire family. Here the failure lies primarily in not first determining the role structure of the family so that time and effort can be invested in the most fruitful direction.

Much the same type of approach is necessary within organizations as well. A health professional who wishes to introduce a change procedure on a particular unit may get the agreement of some staff, but fail to get the change accepted by the entire unit. This may be due to the failure to examine the structure of the unit first, in order to determine who the gatekeeper for that unit is.

COMMUNICATION STRUCTURES

Communication between persons tends to be structured in various ways. Even within a conversation, we can readily note aspects of the communication structure that is involved.

> Head Nurse Fields, with some fifteen years of experience behind her, addresses all the other nurses on her unit by their first name, except when in the presence of patients; then, she addresses them by their last name—e.g., Riley. She prefers to be addressed always by her title and last name: Mrs. Fields. When she speaks with the doctors, however, she uses their title and last name under all circumstances; she would never think of calling a doctor by his or her first name, even in private, in spite of the difference in their ages and years of experience.

The way we address others, using their first name, their last name, or their title and last name—where Dr. and Mrs. are examples of titles—is an aspect of the structure of communication within a conversation that we all employ (e.g., Ervin-Tripp, 1969). In the example, we note several informative aspects of this structure. For example, we see that the head nurse addresses the other nurses on her unit by their first names (when not in the patients' presence), but expects to be referred to by her own title and last name under all circumstances. The form of address exchanged by two or more persons reveals something about the status relationships that exist between them. Research (e.g., Brown & Ford, 1961; Brown & Gilman, 1960) has shown that status equals exchange first names or exchange last names without titles (e.g., Hi, Riley; Hi, Fields), whereas status unequals differ in the structure of their communications: those in status-superior positions expect to be addressed with title and last name while addressing status inferiors by their first name.

Another structural feature revealed in the example involves the head nurse's use of title and last name when addressing the doctors. Even though their experience may be far less than hers, they represent status superiority within the hospital situation. This is reflected in the structure of communication used to address them. Finally, the head nurse does not use first names when addressing the other nurses on her unit if patients are present. This also reflects an aspect of the communication structure involved. Patients fall outside the hospital's status system, but are dealt with in more formal, impersonal ways; thus she feels that it is not appropriate for them to hear the less formal, more personal use of first names. We consider further aspects of communication in Chapter 9.

Networks

Communication structures within groups involve the patterns of communication that take place within the group. The observer of communication will note that not everyone speaks to everyone else, nor, as the illustrative case indicates, not everyone uses the same forms (e.g., of address) when communicating to others. There are patterned flows to the communication that takes place; we can literally see channels that are open to communication and channels that are closed.

The experimental laboratory permits us to intentionally create these various channels of communication in order to study their effects (e.g., Bavelas, 1950; Leavitt, 1958). An example of three such channels in a five-person group is presented in Figure 3–1.

Figure 3–1 illustrates three arrangements of communication that are possible within this five-person group. The circle describes a communication structure in which messages are readily communicated around to everyone. In the chain, messages eventually get around to everyone but there are several intervening steps to be crossed. In the wheel, messages get around but only by passing through the most central position, in this example, the head nurse.

Centrality.   This is one of the key structural features of communication networks such as those illustrated. In the wheel, the most highly central position is the head nurse. In the chain, the doctor and the LPN both occupy the least central positions, being the farthest removed from ready communication with other members of the group.

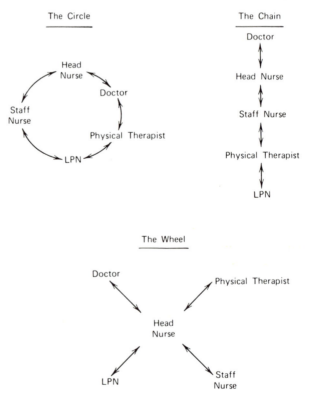

Figure 3-1. Three sample communication structures within groups.

In the circle, all persons are equally central, being the same distance from everyone else.

Research with *simple* laboratory tasks (Leavitt, 1958) has shown that the wheel is the most efficient arrangement for simple problem solving; the chain is next and the circle is the least efficient. However, as the complexity of the task increases, especially as it requires decision making and the evaluation of alternatives, then the circle proves to be the most efficient structure (e.g., Smith, 1951). In fact, with a complex group task, the wheel may be the least efficient, producing the worst decisions if the central person is not very capable or if the peripheral members with good ideas never get a chance to have them evaluated by others in their group. Research (Leavitt, 1958) has also shown that with simple tasks, group morale and a sense of satisfaction is highest in the circle, where all are equally involved, and least high in the wheel, where one member's centrality dominates and leaves the others out of the picture.

While most "real" groups do not appear to be as rigidly structured as those represented in Figure 3–1, there are sufficient parallels to warrant our careful consideration. Persons occupying different positions within a group may indeed never communicate directly with one another; they may always communicate through an intermediary. Or the group's leader may arrange things so that only he or she gains access to all the information needed for decision making, keeping the others more or less in the dark as in the wheel-type structure. Under such circumstances, the competence of this most central person can significantly affect the group's efficiency. For example, a less competent leader can harm the group more when he or she occupies the most central position and thereby receives and evaluates all information and then hands down decisions (see Hyrcenko & Minton, 1974 for a relevant example). In addition, such a highly centralized arrangement does not give others the opportunity to provide checks and balances on their own or on others' suggestions. The burden is put entirely on the leader's shoulders. We return to this theme in the chapter on leadership (Chapter 10).

Although the structures in Figure 3–1 may appear to be rather rigid, they are often reflected in actual groups, especially within organizations such as hospitals and especially as such groups bring together persons of differing social standing. Even less formal groups, including primary groups (e.g., families and informal work teams) have a discernible communication structure. Recall that a structure exists when-

ever we are able to note a pattern of communication that has some stability and continuity even when the persons are exchanged.

ATTRACTION STRUCTURES

Let us suppose that members of a group are asked to name several
people in their group that they most like or feel most friendly toward.
Let us further suppose that these answers are tallied and the results
represented in a diagram. Figure 3–2 provides one possible arrangement of "liking" choices for a group. The circles with initials represent
members of the group. The arrows represent directions of choosing:
e.g., KL→ML means that KL lists ML as one of his or her most liked
persons.

Figure 3–2 indicates several interesting structural features based
on "liking" or attraction. First we note that one person, SN, appears to
be what Moreno (1951; 1953) has called a *sociometric star*. This is a person who occupies a central position in terms of being chosen as most
liked by most of the others in the group. An unchosen person, or
sociometric isolate, in this diagram is represented by MR. Though MR
chooses one other, he or she is unchosen by anyone else in the group.

We can notice another feature of this group's attraction structure.
Several choices are *mutual*, suggesting a pairing of members into
subgroups: e.g., SN and FE; SN and RS; NV and HL. We also notice,
however, that many choices are not reciprocated: e.g., PG is chosen by
HL but does not reciprocate the choice; KL is chosen by PR but does
not reciprocate. Finally, we can note the existence of *pathways* through
the liking structure; these pathways link persons together through

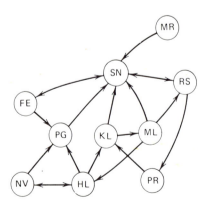

Figure 3-2. The attraction structure of a group.

liked intermediaries: e.g., PR chooses KL who chooses SN who chooses RS who chooses PR. We have other pathways which unlike this circular one, do not return to their point of origin: e.g., HL chooses KL, who chooses SN.

Knowing the attraction structure of a group can provide us with some important information about that group: the morale and level of satisfaction of certain individuals; the alienation of other individuals; the probable pattern and flow of communication within the group; the power and influence structure of the group. Sociometric stars tend to be more satisfied and isolates more alienated. Communication tends to follow the attraction structure: persons linked by liking relationship tend to communicate more with one another. Furthermore, information that enters the group from the outside is likely to flow along the liking pathways. For example, getting some information to NV can result in its flow to HL and PG. From those two, the information branches throughout much of the group. Finally, there tends to be a relation between liking and influence; persons who are well-liked tend to be more influential within the groups than isolates. Thus, knowing the attraction structure of the group can prove informative about its influence structure as well.

Another component of the attraction structure that is relevant involves the degree of reciprocation or nonreciprocation that characterizes an entire group. Where many group members choose others but are not chosen by them in return, we can expect problems of group morale, cohesiveness, and effectiveness in coordinated work. In such a group, people may not perceive one another very clearly; they may send out liking but fail to note that it is not reciprocated; they may feel they have a good relationship with others in their group only to realize one day that this is a faulty perception. This can be damaging to individual self-esteem as well as to group morale.

POWER STRUCTURES

Most groups, including both formal and informal, both primary and secondary, can be characterized by their structures of power, influence, and authority. Families, for example, although defined as primary groups, have their own characteristic power structures. A traditional family is defined in terms of a rather distinct power hierarchy, with the father heading the household and the wife and children "lower" in power. The less traditional, more contemporary family is also characterized by its power structure; in this case, the structure reveals greater equality between husband and wife than in the traditional family. In addition, in many household matters, this modern family form may give children near equality in decision-making influence with the parents.

Other informal groups also have a structure of power, although it may be one that shifts about more than in traditional family groups or in more formally structured groups. Think of some informal groups in which you are a member. Whose decisions seem to carry the most weight when you are all deciding about something to do together? Who is listened to most? Which members elicit the most attentiveness from the others when they speak? Which members elicit the least attention? These are all questions whose answers can help reveal the structure of power and influence within even informal groups.

Within more formal groups, the structuring of power and influence tends to be relatively stable and relatively well-known by all the participants. An investigation reported by Zander, Cohen, and Stotland in 1957, for example, studied the power structure among mental health teams composed of psychiatrists, psychologists, and psychiatric social workers. Their data indicate the not-too-surprising fact that all groups recognize a pecking order with the psychiatrists on top, the psychologists next, and the social workers third. And there was substantial agreement within each group as to this relative ranking in terms of power and influence.

Needless to say, any organization composed of highly trained specialists, each carrying out specific duties involved with patient diagnosis and care, has a relatively stable power structure that varies by profession (e.g., doctors have more authority than RNs), by position within profession (supervisor has more authority than staff); and even by such variables as sex within profession (e.g., males tend to be higher in power and authority than females even within the same profession, even though this too is changing); and prestige outside the organization (e.g., doctors with national reputations tend to gain greater power within the organization than other doctors).

Lest the incorrect picture emerge, we should note that a power structure for a group need not indicate one-way influence. That is, once we have mapped out the hierarchy of power and influence of a group, this mapping does not mean that the position on top has license to do whatever he or she pleases, giving influence and exercising authority but receiving little in return. As we will note in more detail in Chapter 10, the exercise of power is a two-way street; the successful use of power requires an evaluation of factors that resist its acceptance as well. Thus, knowing the power structure of a group does not necessarily inform us about how successful that group is; nor are we informed about how successful the person with the most power is in getting the things accomplished that he or she wishes. But knowing the structure of power and authority of a group does reveal a great deal that we must know if we are to work effectively with the group. Since power and authority overlap so extensively with issues of leadership, we will leave a further discussion of these issues to Chapter 10.

SUMMARY AND CONCLUSIONS

The chapter has dealt with the structural aspects of groups. Structure refers to ordered arrangements that constrain behavior and that provide it with a constancy and stability. Structure is a property of groups and relationships that exists relatively independently of the particular individuals who are involved. Thus, for example, we noted that a group may have a tall (i.e., hierarchical) or a flat (i.e., egalitarian) leadership and power structure that exists as a property of the group separate from the personalities of particular members. We examined several important structural features of groups, including role structures, communication structures, attraction structures, and power structures.

IMPLICATIONS FOR PRACTICE

Several implications for practice were noted throughout this chapter. The one major theme that emerges, however, bears repetition and careful consideration. For the most part, all of us tend to make psychological or individualistic analyses of the causes of behavior. That is, when we try to understand why someone behaves as he or she does, we frequently open our search for an answer by looking for something within the individual person. Often, we search for something within the individual's psychological makeup that helps explain why they did what they did. For example, we notice that the head nurse is short-tempered and ill-humored, a rather unpleasant person. Why? Typically, our answers search for something about her personality that makes her that way.

   The important theme of this chapter, however, argues that we must conduct our search in another way as well. The concept of group structure suggests that people's behavior is regulated and constrained and becomes regularized and stable, *not* entirely by virtue of something about their personality, but by virtue of something about the structural arrangement in which they are located. In other words, as an alternative to an individualistic, psychological analysis we can search for more situational analyses of the behavior we are trying to understand. The head nurse's short-tempered and unpleasant manner therefore may not be simply a function of her personality; it may be a derivative of the kind of organizational or role structure in which she is located. To put this in another way, *anyone* put in her same position would soon become ill-tempered and unpleasant.

Having noted that a structural interpretation and analysis is an important alternative to an individual, psychological analysis, we must next note the implication of this alternative for our practice. Structural changes rather than personality changes may be required to alleviate strain and increase effectiveness. In other words, a change in personnel may not produce greater effectiveness if the source of the problem is structural. New personnel will soon get trapped by the same structural arrangements and suffer the same consequences. We could continue to change people and never find the solution if the critical source of the difficulty is structural.

Practitioners of group process must be sensitive to this structural analysis of behavior. They must be aware of the various kinds of group structure that exist (e.g., role, communication, attraction, and power) and of the ways in which these structures influence both individual and group behavior. For example, a particular communication structure called the wheel may prove highly alienating to individuals and may result in low group morale. Morale can be improved and individual alienation lessened by an intervention that effects a change in the communication structure rather than by an intervention plan that ignores this critical structural property.

A structural rather than a purely individualistic analysis of a group or organizational issue (e.g., a problem or difficulty such as low morale, poor team effectiveness, etc.) serves another important practical function as well. When individual analyses are predominant, we not only blame individuals for their problem, but also hold them responsible for doing something to change it. It is then easy for such people to feel guilty, as if they have failed; they blame themselves; self-esteem is lowered, and they may experience frustration and despair as they continue to duplicate failure. A structural analysis suggests that the individual's woes may not be entirely of his or her own making; that is, a person may be caught in a situation that would make anyone feel troubled and disturbed. By expanding the locus of our understanding, therefore, we not only reformulate our conception of a proper intervention strategy (i.e., structural rather than psychological) but also help alleviate the individual from the full burden of guilt and consequent loss of self-esteem.

For example, the newly graduated RN who faces her first job may undergo a series of experiences that are common to all RNs who work within particular kinds of hospital structure. Her sense of failure and depression may be common to all in her position and not simply a response that is unique to her alone. A structural analysis can thereby help her cope better with the reality of her situation; it can help her direct her attention toward the structures that are at fault rather than getting caught up in self-blame, despair, and depression.

It is often the health professional who must make a structural analysis available as an alternative to the individual, the group, or the organization, so that energies can be directed away from self-blame and toward a more appropriate source. This redirection, in turn, can facilitate effective coping with the real issue. But before the practitioner can facilitate this redirection, he or she must first be able to understand what a structural analysis means. And this has been the purpose of this chapter.

4

Group Norms and Standards

*A*ll groups—formal and informal, primary and secondary—have sets of standards for the behavior, attitudes, and even the perceptions of their members. These standards are called the *norms* of the group: shared expectations for what is appropriate and inappropriate behavior, what members should and shouldn't do. All groups not only have norms—they also have mechanisms whereby conformity to these norms is accomplished, ways in which group pressures are brought to bear on members who stray too far from the group's norms.

The *content* of the norms tends to vary from group to group, as does the degree to which the norms are *explicit* or *implicit*. Groups also vary in the form which normative pressures take, in the intensity of these pressures, and in the targets of these normative pressures: i.e., who in the group is permitted more or less leeway in following the norms.

Extensity

There are some groups in which the content of the norms cover all aspects of the members' lives. Membership in some religious groups, for example, carries along with it expectations for nearly all behaviors and attitudes that members should have. The content of such norms, thus, is extensive, directing members' manner of dress, their private behavior, their public attitudes and conduct, and so forth. On the other hand, occupational groups, especially in complex societies, tend to emphasize normative content that centers more on job-related issues. Members' private lives are usually not under the direction of occupational group norms; rather, such behavior tends to be encompassed by the norms of people's informal, family, and friendship groups.

Medical and health specialties often fomulate group norms for members that extend widely, encompassing the members' private lives. These norms often involve ethical issues, outlining behaviors that health professionals should and should not engage in within their professional practice as well as their private lives. Medical and other health professionals are also typically under wide-ranging normative pressure to be willing to sacrifice much of their own personal and private life (especially time) to their profession. Teachers, for example, may be expected to put in a work week of generally defined and limited hours; it is usually considered appropriate for them to resist efforts to cut into their personal time. Health professionals, however, typically have less personal time and greater expectations to be on call and available; they can properly make some efforts to protect their private moments, but in general, normative expecations allow them less free time than other occupational groups.

Within the typical work group or health professional team, the content of group norms typically focuses on work-related issues: e.g., the appropriate tasks for the members; the ways members interact with one another both on and off the job; the way patients are dealt with; the kinds of clothing that should and shouldn't be worn; the perspectives on treatment; the extent of openness and trust among members; the formality or informality of relationships within the group; the type of leadership style legitimate for the group; and so forth.

Explicitness

In noting that norms may be explicit or implicit, we wish to call attention to the fact that some groups have stated an explicit set of guidelines for proper member behavior; at times, these are presented to new members who are to learn them as part of their induction into the group. Other groups, though having many norms and standards for members' behavior, are much less explicit about these. These norms appear as an implicit, shared understanding that members have about what is and what is not appropriate behavior. Even groups with a set of very explicit norms also tend to have many implicit understandings. Thus a new member may learn the explicit set of rules rather readily, but may require much additional time before he or she can grasp these implicit understandings. A new nurse, for example, may violate the implicit norms of her team by asking too many questions; though this is never stated as an explicit group norm, in time she learns that question-asking is a behavior that this team regulates and feels should be kept to a minimum.

One way to determine the norms of a group is to ask the members (including oneself as a member), "What is considered appropriate and what is considered inappropriate behavior for members of this group?" For example, if a member is late for a meeting (or in a family, if someone arrives late to dinner), would that be considered appropriate or inappropriate? Are there rules or opinions about being on time in this group? In conducting even so simple an exercise, it may be surprising to discover the number of norms that exist within any one group, the content that is covered by these norms, and the degree to which they are explicit.

Conformity

Conformity to norms, while expected in all groups, is handled differently in different groups. Even within the same group, normative pressures (i.e., group pressures to conform to the norm) are handled differently for different members. Groups have several ways to achieve conformity to norms. For the most part, other than using threatened or actual physical restraint or punishment—an approach that characterizes some families, some classrooms, some military and athletic groups, and some institutionalized groups—the more usual approaches involve verbal influence, including praising or reproaching members, and rejection, even to the point of actual ostracism from the group.

The potency of most norms, however, is their quality of being understood without members always having to test them out and receive punishment. Conformity to group norms becomes rewarding in itself to the group's members. They feel good about behaving in ways that are considered appropriate by their group and feel guilt or shame when behaving inappropriately. Members are rewarded by the acceptance of their fellow members when they follow norms; often, higher prestige and status within the group hinges on members' behaving in ways that live up to the group's standards.

For example, on a particular team, there is an unspoken but shared norm regarding innovation in developing care plans for patients. A student who is innovative in giving and in recommending care is praised by other team members; his or her status rises within the group and the level of acceptance by others is increased. Deviancy does not earn much esteem from fellow members. Much conformity to group norms occurs without actual punishment ever having to be undertaken.

Idiosyncrasy Credit

Not all members are subjected to the same kinds of normative pressure or sanction for having violated the norms. Although the research on this point is not completely firm in its conclusions, there are indications that persons of higher status within a group can deviate from norms with relative impunity as compared with members of lesser status. Coming in late for dinner, for example, may bring harsh punishment for a child but little repercussion for the father. Or the chairperson who has called the group together may arrive late with little punishment whereas anyone arriving after that person may be considered late and treated accordingly. In most medical settings, a physician can arrive late to a scheduled meeting with relative impunity; on the other hand, a student or a staff nurse arriving late meets with disapproval or even direct punishment.

Hollander (1958; 1961) introduced the concept of *idiosyncrasy credit* to refer to one aspect of this issue. He suggested that members who dutifully follow their group's norms not only earn higher prestige within the group as examples of what a "good" member is but also build up a credit against future deviance: these are termed idiosyncrasy credits. In this view, a person with a high "credit rating" can behave idiosyncratically in violation of group norms, with relative impunity. When the credit runs out, however, conformity to group standards is again expected. Members who are new to a group or who have never built up much credit are those most likely to be sanctioned for any departures from appropriate behavior.

If a person were to adopt this concept as a self-conscious policy for behavior, then he or she would spend some initial time in a new group building up credits by conforming fully to group norms. These early credits could then be spent later. The staff nurse who always shows up at meetings on time and in other ways earns a reputation as a good group member may gain greater leeway than the person who has never built up credits in the first place.

Visibility and Pressure

Groups and roles within groups often vary in the degree to which behaviors are open to observation and evaluation by other members or outsiders. This describes the *visibility* of the group or role. A role with high visibility is one in which the person's performance is open to the scrutiny and evaluation of others. With low visibility, one cannot be evaluated as readily by others, and thus conformity to group norms is less easily determined. Visibility is related to group norms and normative pressures; less visibility permits greater deviation from normative expectations. Basically, those behaviors that are more open to the surveillance and evaluation of others permit less leeway for deviation from group norms when compared with behaviors that are low in their visibility. Arriving late for a meeting is a behavior of high visibility and thus is readily open to sanctions. The job attitude a person has, however, tends to be of lesser visibility. Even though group norms may demand that members all share a high level of enthusiasm for their work, any member can feel little enthusiasm without being the recipient of group sanctions for this "invisible" deviant attitude. Of course, if the attitude leaks into a public display or obvious discontent and low motivation, then sanctions are likely.

THE FUNCTION OF NORMS AND NORMATIVE PRESSURES

Norms do not simply arise within groups nor do pressures to conform to these norms simply evolve for the sake of making life more troublesome for members who would be free spirits. Analysts of group process have suggested several important functions served by norms and normative pressures.

Task Functions

In the first place, a hypothetical, purely fictional group that sought to function without any normative regulation of members' behavior would give meaning to the idea of chaos. One critical function that norms serve is to permit groups to function in relatively coordinated ways in the accomplishment of their tasks and goals. We would expect, therefore, that the most explicit statement of norms and the greatest pressure for conformity to such norms would converge around the task functions of goal attainment, at least in groups for which task achievement is the critical purpose for existence. Groups that are organized around more social functions, on the other hand, may play down goal achievement and emphasize norms that deal with members' interpersonal styles, openness, friendliness, compatibility, and so forth.

Maintenance Functions

A second function which norms and normative pressures serve falls more directly in the group maintenance area. Not all groups will emphasize maintenance issues, but the problem of group maintenance exists whenever two or more persons convene for whatever purpose. Thus we would expect to find norms developing around maintenance issues such as attendance at group meetings, standards about how disagreements are to be expressed and resolved, behaviors involving conflict and its resolution, standards involving members' personal relations, and so forth.

Social Reality Functions

A critical third function that group norms and normative pressures serve involves what have been called *social reality functions* (Festinger, 1954; Schachter, 1951). Most of the issues with which each of us deal in our daily lives at work and elsewhere confront us with matters that involve the interpretation of fact. In measuring blood pressure, for example, the factual matter involves the reading on the gauge. This is something that we can determine relatively independently of others and with little interpretation required. However, the decision about what that reading means and what the next step in the diagnostic procedure should be, begins to converge on matters of interpretation. We choose the word "interpretation" rather than "opinion" in order to emphasize that the arena of social reality is not simply one of opinion about this or that matter; rather, social reality pertains to the interpretation that persons make of even hard facts and hard data. Thus, interpretation extends throughout all facets of our living and practice.

In matters of interpretation, judgments must be made regarding the status of reality. The gauge reads 120/80, but what does this mean? The reality in such interpretative matters is embedded in social contexts; thus it is referred to as a social reality as distinct from the sheer physical realtiy of the reading on the gauge. To say that reality is social is to note that the evaluation of its truth or falsity is social; that is, it depends on agreements of interpretation rendered by others with whom we associate, including others who publish in scholarly journals and whose analyses become accepted as facts.

Perceptual Facts.   To say that reality is social is to emphasize the group processes that are involved in constituting and creating what we take to be real, true, and valid (e.g., Berger & Luckman, 1966). Much laboratory research in social psychology has been concerned with examining how group norms develop in the service of providing persons with a sense of a shared social reality, even in matters that ostensibly appear not to require an extensive interpretation. The early work of Asch, for example (1952), showed how persons would actually change their own perception or verbal reports about the length of a line presented to them after they heard the estimate provided by other members of their group. Thus members were influenced to see or to report their own judgment of the line's length so as not to depart too much from the estimates given by others in their group. Deutsch and Gerard (1955) later demonstrated that the more the individuals felt themselves to be members of a group—that is, the more interdependent they were—the more extensive was the effect of the group's normative judgments on the individual's own estimates.

Frame of Reference.   In more ambiguous settings, others (e.g., Sherif, 1935) have demonstrated how groups provide a judgmental frame of reference or norm within which members come to evaluate the status of reality. In Sherif's work, the reality involved the distance a point of light apparently moved in a darkened room. Over a period of some time together, groups developed a standard for judging this distance; once a standard emerged, it provided the framework within which members came to perceive the light's movement. For example, in one group the consensus developed that the light was moving somewhere in the range of 2 to 5 inches. This served as a framework within which individuals came to make their own assessments of its movement. Thus, a member would report his or her judgment somewhere within that 2 to 5-inch standard; to report something smaller or greater than that range would be to deviate from the group's standard or norm of judgment regarding the light's movement. In similar fashion, group norms provide the frame of reference within which we make our own judgments about social reality.

Resistance.   In the many critical matters of social reality, the touchstone by which we gauge our own interpretations about what is and what is not correct, true, or real is given by the groups to which we belong or whose views we have come to accept as offering us a valid perspective (e.g., Newcomb, 1958; 1961; Newcomb et al., 1967). Many group norms thereby offer the individual social definitions and interpretations of reality. Normative pressures involve ways of dealing with potentially threatening challenges to these shared definitions of reality. Members who stray too far from the group's norms cast doubt on the validity of the interpretations that are used to understand social reality. It is difficult to be open and hospitable to such challenges. Not surprisingly, some of the strongest normative pressures are brought to bear whenever the deviation pertains to this social reality function.

For example, the resistance of a team health professionals to a new procedure or technique often involves the implication that adherents to the old way are thereby incorrect or misguided in their views regarding diagnosis or patient care. New discoveries that open old practices to doubt are often met with resistance and even rejection.

Resistance to innovation can occur when a new practice involves something as simple and noncontroversial as the use of a team approach in the treatment of selected surgical patients. For instance, Mrs. Watts will require colostomy surgery. Should a rehabilitation team of health professionals consisting of a physician, a nurse-specialist, a nutritionist, a physical therapist, a psychologist, and a social worker be developed to work with Mrs. Watts and her family throughout the surgical procedure and afterward? In this case, resistance may develop around the very idea of a team approach.

Some medical specialists may doubt that a team approach is appropriate in this case. In their view, she will undergo surgery and will only require a few follow-up visits. The idea of a team of health professionals to develop and carry out a treatment plan for her and her family is the kind of innovation that may meet resistance. As we probe the basis of this resistance, we realize that it implies something about the validity of the old practice: that is, the implication is that a team approach is necessary because the old way is not satisfactory. And this implication is a clear threat to those with vested interests in the old ways of practice; thus, much of their resistance is based on the threats to their concepts of what medical reality in the treatment of cancer is all about.

But it need not be a new procedure or a new discovery. A new group member may bring with her the practices of her former groups and meet great resistance from the new group: "We don't do things that way around here."

Nurse Arlington has attended several human sexuality workshops and is concerned with the sexuality issues that are involved in nursing and medical practice. In an effort to determine more about these issues, she begins to make some informal inquiries of her co-workers on her new job at City Hospital. The group on her former unit and her sexuality training groups all had norms in which the discussion of sexuality was a rather routine matter; people were encouraged to talk openly and nondefensively about sexual feelings, impulses, ideas, practices, myths, and so forth as they were relevant to patient care. Nurse Arlington believes nothing is unusual, therefore, about making the same kind of inquiries on her new job. She is quite mistaken. Although no one directly approaches her and says, "Those questions are not appropriate around here" (another norm of this new group involves never confronting others directly with disagreements) she is made to realize in any number of indirect ways that her questions are a violation of her new group's standards.

As we try to understand the basis for the group's resistance to Nurse Arlington's questioning, we discover the social reality function that underlies their norms against uncovering issues of sexuality.

The group as a whole does not resist Nurse Arlington's questioning because it pertains to sexual issues, although some individual members may do so. More significantly, the resistance occurs because the content falls outside the group's definition of what is relevant (i.e., real, true, valid, correct) for medical and nursing practice. The group has shared definitions of nursing and medical practice that excludes issues of sexuality in much the same way that astrological or political issues are excluded from their definitions of social reality relevent to health care.

Nurse Arlington's questioning about sexuality casts doubt upon the groups' exclusion of what they may suspect to be an important concern to their practice but one which thus far they have refused to confront. Their resistance reflects the problems that including her ideas into their own analysis would entail: e.g., everyone would have to become familiar with human sexuality and its relation to their practice as health care professionals; they might even have to rethink their own practices and dramatically revise some of their procedures.

The Social Basis of Reality.   Of all the functions that norms and normative pressures serve, the social reality function is perhaps one of the most complex and least understood by most practitioners. Basically, we must realize that much of what we know and accept to be true and valid is socially determined. We accept as matters of fact many matters of social interpretation. We search for those groups that provide confirmation for our ways of interpretating and knowing reality; we pressure those whose alternative interpretations challenge our own; we ask them to leave or to be quiet so that we need not open up our own views of reality to excessive doubt. All groups have evolved their own normative definitions and interpretations of reality; and all groups bring pressures to bear on members to remain within the fold of their views.

Not too surprisingly, people leave groups when competing perspectives on social reality force them to meet the challenge by adopting another group's analysis. Not surprisingly, people join groups whose points of view mesh relatively closely with their own. And not surprisingly, we all participate in bringing normative pressures to bear on those who seem to violate our collective sense of the right and proper reality. In that interpretative issues pervade all of our practice—that is, no matter how factual the base of our practice, the context of meaning within which to interpret those facts is socially rooted—the social reality function of group norms and normative pressures likewise pervades much of what we do.

INTENSITY OF NORMATIVE PRESSURES

Research (e.g., Schachter, 1951) has suggested two important factors that affect the intensity of the pressures for members to adopt and follow group norms: *relevance* and *cohesiveness*.

Relevance

Relevance refers to the idea that group norms can vary in their importance to a group's task functions, its maintenance functions, or its social reality functions. The greater the relevance of the norm to any of these functions, the greater will be the pressure on members to follow that norm. For example, if the task of a group is to meet and plan a curriculum for in-service training, group norms that involve the way members should dress at the meetings would appear less relevant to that task and thus less likely to involve normative pressures than matters more central to the task at hand: e.g., how competing philosophies of nursing will be expressed and resolved by the group. We are all aware, however, of seemingly irrelevant matters that can become of great concern to a group. Issues of social reality and group maintenance have a way of encompassing many content areas. The way a member dresses for a curriculum committee meeting, for example, may be "read" by the group leader as a sign of commitment to the group or as rejection of the group and its goals. Thus, even clothing might be considered highly relevant. In general, however, once we have determined areas and functions that are of high and low relevance to a particular group, then we can know what behaviors are most and least likely to receive normative pressures. And much of this determination is based on the purposes and goals of the group.

Cohesiveness

We previously encountered the concept of cohesiveness in Chapter 2; we saw that it refers to the members' attraction to their group. This attraction can be based on several things (Cartwright & Zander, 1968):

—Attraction to the *members* of the group
—Attraction to the *task* of the group
—Attraction to the *goals and ideals* of the group

Whatever its source, however, a highly cohesive group is one in which members are highly attracted to remain in the group; a group having low cohesiveness is one in which the members are minimally attracted to the group.

Cohesiveness is related to normative pressures in a rather straightforward way: the more cohesive the group, the greater the normative pressures (see Festinger et al., 1950, for a classic study of this effect). When we focus on an individual member of the group, the same relationship holds; the more attracted a particular member is to his or her group, the more will that person be responsive to normative pressures. Essentially, the more cohesive the group, the more its members are attracted to their membership and want the group to remain together as a group; under these conditions, members give and receive more pressure to follow group norms than do less cohesive groups. In the latter groups, with minimal attraction to membership and little concern for the group as a whole, there is little pressure either given or received to follow group norms.

Combining both relevance and cohesiveness, we would expect groups that are highly cohesive to bring the greatest normative pressures to bear on members for issues that are most relevant and central to the group's functioning. The combination of high cohesiveness and high relevance should produce the greatest pressures; the combination of low cohesiveness and low relevance should produce the least pressure for normative conformity. Often, what seems to be chaotic and confused group functioning and little coordination among the members reflects this very condition of low cohesiveness and low relevance. Research reported by Schachter (1951) has provided some valuable support for the joint effects of relevance and cohesiveness; other investigators have substantially confirmed the connection between a group's level of cohesiveness and the pressures on members to follow group norms (Cartwright & Zander, 1968, provide a useful discussion of some of this work).

IMPLICATIONS FOR PRACTICE: THE IMPORTANCE OF UNDERSTANDING GROUP NORMS

Implied throughout our discussion of group norms and normative pressures are reasons why the student of group process would benefit from a knowledge of these concepts. Let us, however, confront the practical issue more directly. Several writers about group process help sharpen our discussion of the practical issues involved.

Lewin's Analysis

In Chapter 1, we introduced some of Lewin's ideas about the role of group processes in behavior maintenance and change. His analysis indicates that a group's norms and standards are *the* critical element in both maintaining an individual's existing behaviors and attitudes and in providing the context for changing them. To understand an individual's health practices, for example, we need to understand the norms of the groups to which that individual belongs or to which he or she aspires to belong (i.e., the person's reference groups). Furthermore, to implement a program of change in that individual's health practices, we would have to effect a change in the norms of those same groups or provide the individual with group contexts whose norms support a more desirable set of health practices. In other words, we can neither understand an individual's existing behaviors and attitudes nor hope to change them without an understanding of the normative processes that are involved.

Argyris' Analysis

While we attach the name of Argyris to this perspective, many others have reached a similar conclusion: often it is the norms of groups that work to prevent the group's effectiveness. Thus, to increase group effectiveness, diagnosing normative patterns and working to change them (e.g., Lieberman et al., 1973) is often required. Argyris bases his conclusions on the results of a large-scale investigation of actual problem-solving and decision-making groups in business and industry, the government, universities, and other types of organizations (see Argyris, 1969). His data suggested that the dominant pattern of norms that characterized most of these groups (he referred to this as Pattern A) involved: (a) being generally closed to other members' ideas but especially their feelings; (b) being generally distrustful of others; (c) refusing to experiment with alternative ideas or ways of doing things; (d) generally going along with existing norms, valuing conformity to these norms, and trying not to rock the boat. Let us quote Argyris' conclusions about groups characterized by this normative pattern:

> The consequences of Pattern A behavior were relatively ineffective interpersonal relationships and ineffective problem solving of task issues that were important and loaded with feelings. When solutions were achieved, they did not tend to be lasting ones. The problems therefore seemed to recur continually. Finally, members seemed to be blind to the negative impact that they tended to have on others (partially because it violated the norms to give such feedback); they were accurately aware of the impact others have upon them, but careful not to communicate this impact openly or directly. (pp. 898–899)

In that Pattern A seems to predominate in the groups that Argyris has studied and clearly to predominate in most groups of health professionals, the group process practitioner faces a real challenge to his or her practice. What we have noted is that a group's norms can thwart effective group practice; and that the typical normative pattern is one that generally produces ineffective problem solving. The practitioner must therefore work to evaluate and change group norms in order to have any hope for accomplishing effective group process; and this is nowhere more true than in the health professions.

The health team dealing with the Watts family is a good case in point. If it were to function according to the Pattern A description, then we would expect to find the following things occur:

1. Each specialist on the team would push his or her own point of view and generally be closed to hearing or responding to the views and ideas of other members.

2. Feelings concerning the way the group was functioning or the effectiveness of its treatment plan would never be openly expressed or examined; therefore people on the team would never really know how anyone else felt about what they were supposedly doing together.

3. Team members would act in generally distrustful ways toward one another; they would not reveal ideas and opinions to others if they felt that they would not gain acceptance; they would be wary of one another, and act in polite but distant ways.

4. The possibilities for engaging in innovative treatment plans would be minimized because members felt it was neither appropriate nor wise to experiment with new ideas; the tendency would be for the team to continue to tread the old pathways and not venture into anything new or different.

5. Members would most highly value conforming with existing group norms; in particular, they would be likely to value going along with the medical doctor who heads the team, not wishing to seriously question or challenge his or her ideas, seeing any such challenges as rocking the boat.

It is highly doubtful that a group governed by such norms could function effectively as a team to provide excellent care to Mrs. Watts and her family. To function effectively, this team would have to examine the norms that members had created together and work toward restructuring those very norms that thwart effective team practice. While this is not an easy process, it is a realistic and possible process; it is one of which the practitioner must be mindful, especially as team practice becomes increasingly a model for health care.

Groupthink and the Conflict Perspective

Based on his examination of high-level governmental decision-making groups, Janis (1973) introduced the term *groupthink* to describe a normative pattern similar in many respects to Argyris' Pattern A. Groupthink refers to the tendency within many groups to eschew conflict and adopt a normative pattern in which the good group member is loyal to the group's leader and other members, never really challenging or seriously doubting the leader's or the group's wisdom in matters of decision making. Groupthink, like Pattern A norms, typically leads to ineffective group functioning. Alternatives are never seriously considered by the group; members fear that to bring up a different possibility is to openly challenge the serene loyalty that is normatively demanded. Members follow groupthink norms, refusing to provide the kinds of seriously probing questions that all decision-making groups need in developing and testing out their proposals before enacting them as policy. We consider groupthink again in Chapter 10.

Researchers, such as Maier and his several colleagues, have provided further perspective on this important function; effective group problem solving derives from encouraging openness and conflict within the group rather than from a normative pattern that discourages any open exchange of ideas and points of view (see Maier, 1970). Maier's research data suggest that both leadership style and group norms that converge around conflict avoidance hinder effective group problem solving. We will consider this issue of leadership style in Chapter 10. The normative picture is what concerns us at this point. Clearly, if some degree of conflict of ideas is necessary to effective group problem solving and if excessive loyalty thwarts the introduction of challenges to the existing decisions and alternatives (as with Pattern A or groupthink), then groups characterized by these norms and normative pressures will not be as effective as groups with different norms.

The intimate connection between a group's norms and its effectiveness is sufficiently great to warrant our concern with norms and normative pressures as a matter of urgent practicality. To be able to recognize a group's normative status is important to any student of group process or for that matter, any individuals for whom group process enters as a significant component of their practice.

SUMMARY AND CONCLUSIONS

Group norms refer to shared standards for behavior, attitudes, and perception that characterize all kinds of group. The existence of norms gives rise to pressures on members to follow these norms. These pressures vary as a function of the relevance of the norms to the purposes of the group and the cohesiveness of the group. Norms serve task, maintenance, and social reality functions. The analysis of a group's norms and normative pressures is vital to an understanding of group process. Much of what goes on in groups involves the development and transformation of norms and the processes involved in maintaining members' conformity to norms. It is virtually impossible to comprehend individual behavior in a group without an understanding of group norms and how these norms influence members' conceptions of themselves and their daily practice. The intimate connection between a group's effectiveness and its pattern of norms demands that we understand norms and normative pressures if our interest lies in working more effectively in and with groups.

III

Theoretical Background and Perspectives

The mere mention of the word "theory" leads many people to tune out the speaker. They think that theories are either too complex or too abstract to be of any value in their everyday practice. It is true that theories often are complex: they develop abstractions often far removed from our simple and direct observations; and they organize these abstractions into even more general statements. Yet we agree with Kurt Lewin, who stated some years ago that there is nothing as practical as a good theory. Practitioners need good theory before they can participate in good practice. In our view, the theories of group process are best seen as practical guides to understanding and practice.

Functions of Theory

Theories serve three critical functions: they influence (1) what we see and what we consider to be factual data; (2) how we organize and interpret these data; and (3) what we do about it—that is, how we intervene to affect the process. A theory of group process helps focus our attention on certain key aspects of what goes on when people come together and interact in groups. A theory offers us ways of organizing our thinking about what we have seen; it provides us with an intelligible grasp of what is otherwise often a confusing array of apparently disconnected behaviors. And finally, theories of group process are practical guides to intervention and management of the process itself. Without a theory to guide us, we have little basis for knowing how, when, or why to intervene. Thus, theories are vital to our roles as group leaders and organizers.

Common-Sense Theories

Not surprisingly, whatever our formal knowledge of theories may be, all of us employ common-sense theories in our everyday dealings with others. These implicit, personal theories serve the same functions as do formal theories. Our personal theories of group process affect what we see, how we interpret it, and what we do about it. Too often, however, our personal theories are so implicit that we function in the dark with little awareness that we are even using a "theory" to guide us.

> Dr. Anderson, a third-year psychiatric resident, is in charge of an adolescent unit. He has established some highly structured guidelines for the adolescents in his care. He is particularly concerned that each adolescent follow the same schedule of activities and that no deviations be allowed. He and his staff ignore any differences among the adolescents, treating everyone the same. Some of their patients, however, rebel from time to time, rejecting these rigid rules by acting in an unruly, defiant manner. Dr. Anderson and his staff interpret this unruly behavior as symptomatic of the adolescent's psychiatric disturbance and respond by taking away privileges and putting the defiant ones under even more rigid controls.

The incident just described contains all the elements of a theory, even though Dr. Anderson and others on his staff may not realize that they are using a theory to guide their actions in dealing with the adolescents on their unit. The implicit theory, however, guides what they see, how they interpret it, and what they do about it: they attend carefully to behavior that violates specific rules; they interpret this behavior as a symptom of psychiatric disturbance; and they intervene to control it by punishment (i.e., withdrawal of privileges).

What their implicit theory fails to provide them, however, is another view and analysis of the same situation. If their implicit theories could become explicit, they could thereby better understand the bases of their actions and even choose an alternate approach. For example, normal adolescents typically rebel against what appear to be arbitrary rules; they defiantly act out and test rules as a gesture of their evolving independence from adult control. In this alternate view, rebellion is not automatically symptomatic of psychiatric disturbance, but rather may be indicative of normal, healthy growth. The adolescent who is excessively compliant, who dutifully follows all adult rules without question, may be more in need of our concern and attention. Intervening with punishment in circumstances in which growth is taking place, in this alternate view, may serve to thwart growth toward independence and thus not be a desirable intervention.

This case illustrates several points. First, we all operate every day according to personal, usually implicit theories that guide our understanding of and intervention in group process. Second, if these implicit theories became more explicit and open to our scrutiny, we could discard them if we became aware that they had undesirable consequences. Third, we can become more aware of our own implicit theories and thereby correct them only when we confront explicit alternatives. These explicit alternatives, in turn, are basically the major theories that exist within the field of group process. They offer us alternatives to our implicit theories; they help us attend to behaviors that we might not otherwise have seen, to interpret these behaviors in ways we might not otherwise have used, and to intervene in ways that we might not otherwise have considered. All in all, therefore, our study of Chapters 5 to 8 provides us with some helpful and important guidelines to our everyday practice.

Several major theories of group process will be presented. We will be selective and thus will not consider every view that has been offered. Each theory we examine differs in what aspects of group process it emphasizes, what it ignores, how it interprets what it sees, and what recommendations it makes for intervention. It is our hope that a careful consideration of these several theories will give the student a set of alternatives from which to choose rather than one simple approach that is considered to be the "real truth." Each has much to offer us.

Chapter 5 is focused on psychoanalytic theories, which are primarily based on the pioneering work of Freud. These theories emphasize the important role that the unconscious plays in individual, interpersonal, and group behavior. We cannot be satisfied with scanning the surface or stopping our inquiry with a mere analysis of superficial behaviors and actions. In Chapter 5 we are urged to conduct our inquiry below the surface; the unconscious holds the key to understanding behavior. When we turn that key, it unlocks the door to the history of the people involved. Chapter 5 also demonstrates that unconscious matters are not just beyond awareness; they cannot easily enter awareness. We learn that an active *barrier* separates the world of our awareness from the world of our unconscious. Resistance to awareness is a central idea we will discuss in this chapter.

Chapter 6 introduces the symbolic interactionist perspective; its origins are derived from the social psychological and philosophical writings of George Herbert Mead. Unlike the Freudian emphasis on concealed processes taking place beneath surface awareness, the Meadian viewpoint emphasizes those interactions taking place here-and-now. It is concerned with the ways that people jointly establish the meanings that form and guide their interactions together. We learn that what something means does not reside in that something but rather emerges in the course of human interaction. For example, a chair does not intrinsically mean something to sit on; rather, as people relate to that object in terms of its qualities as a seat rather than its potential as a weapon, its familiar meaning (i.e., a seat) emerges. According to the Meadian perspective, no meanings are more important than those involving the concept of identity or self. In this view, group life is understoods as a flowing, living process within which people create, sustain, or undermine their own and others' identities. Even as the meaning of a chair as something to sit on is sustained or transformed within group interaction, so too is the meaning of our own identity and the identities of other people. The symbolic interactionist theory gives a very different perspective on human interaction and group life than we might otherwise adopt.

Chapter 7 takes a third and still different look at group process. Group life is now seen in terms of processes of exchange and equilibrium. The group is treated as a small social system that strives to maintain a state of balance or equilibrium; both its internal and external environments provide ample opportunities to overturn the momentary homeostasis. A kind of organic metaphor becomes the centerpiece of what we call the systems analysis: the group is like an organism that takes in nutrients and eliminates wastes, that strives to maintain a state of equilibrium in spite of changing conditions and circumstances, that is composed of opposing sets of forces and tendencies, and that engages in exchanges with both its external and its internal environments.

Chapter 8 introduces the dimension of time and the concepts of growth and development into the theoretical framework of group process. Unlike a photograph that freezes time, the theories of group development place their emphasis on understanding the ways in which time affects the interpersonal world of group process. Theories that focus on stages or phases of group process are examined in this chapter.

These four theory chapters introduce four key concepts in group process:

1. The unconscious and resistance to its becoming conscious.
2. The creation of meanings and identities as products or outcomes of social interaction and group process.
3. The understanding of the individual member as part of the process governing the pursuit of equilibrium for the whole system.
4. The effects of time on group and individual behavior.

5

Psychoanalytic Approaches:
Unconscious Processes
in Group Behavior

Although we tend to connect the psychoanalytic theories of Freud and his followers with the psychology of individuals, these theories have much to say about groups and interpersonal relations as well. The concept of *transference*, for example, was introduced by Freud in order to explain the otherwise puzzling projections that occurred during the therapy hour with patients (Freud, 1924–1950). According to this concept, patients relate to their therapist *as if* the therapist were a reminder of a person from their past: e.g., their father or mother. They demonstrate deep attachments or harbor deep antipathies toward the therapist. In a sense, patients are believed by Freudians to replay their family drama with the therapist, transferring to him or her their earlier feelings and relationships. This transference makes the therapy itself an interpersonal rather than a purely individual matter. The key to treatment, according to this theory, is for the therapist and patient to examine and work through these transferences. In this sense, therefore, Freud's individual psychology is in truth a group or interpersonal psychology as well.

It was in his relatively brief but important work on group psychology that Freud (1960) set forth the more complex details of his analysis of group process. Not surprisingly, the main focus of the psychoanalytic approach is on unconscious processes and relationships such as those involved in transference. The great lesson that Freud taught us is to examine what lies beneath the apparent surface of conscious life in order to gain a fuller understanding of and appreciation for the complexities of human behavior. In particular, his group psychology was based on understanding members' unconscious relationship to the group's leader; this exemplifies an extension of the transference theme in therapy to the study of normal group process.

THE HIDDEN AGENDA

When we talk about an unconscious process with reference to a group, just what do we mean? Without delving too deeply into the complex matter of trying to locate a group's unconscious, we will introduce the concept of the *hidden agenda* in order to sharpen our focus. Let us assume that whenever persons come together to interact, there are two levels on which that interaction takes place. That is, all group interactions involve two agendas—one conscious, often publicly stated, explicit, and open for everyone to see; the other hidden beneath the surface, implicit, closed from direct public scrutiny and awareness, but emerging nevertheless to influence whatever takes place.

A simple example involves a student in a classroom who asks the teacher a question to which he already knows the answer (Yalom, 1975). On the surface, the stated agenda involves asking a question and obtaining an answer. But beneath the surface there lies another agenda. This becomes apparent when the student corrects the teacher's incorrect answer. Although all the attributes of that hidden agenda may not be known by the observer, it is a pretty good guess that it involves some effort on the part of the student to dominate or assert domination over a public authority figure. That is, the public agenda of asking a question may in this case cover a hidden agenda of attacking or challenging persons in authority.

The concept of the hidden agenda or unconscious group process is important primarily because the surface, observed behavior is not adequate to a complete understanding of the situation. Something more seems to be going on. Often, what we observe on the surface does not make much sense without an explicit concept such as that of the hidden agenda to enrich our understanding. The development of this concept of unconscious processes has emerged from many observations of many groups over a considerable period of time; it is a concept of interpretation that has been tested and typically found worthwhile.

This latter point is important. There is much resistance on the part of the beginning student and on the part of the group itself to the idea that unconscious processes may play a significant role in our behavior. Let us suppose that the teacher of the previous example not only had the suspicion about the student's "hidden agenda item" but also checked it out directly and bluntly with the student: e.g., "Are you asking me a question to which you already know the answer because you are really trying to challenge and attack me?" We would not expect the student to smile and answer, "Yes, that's it!"

Agendas are hidden from the participants as well; thus it is not reasonable to expect that a direct check will readily reveal what are often very deep lying unconscious processes. But such concepts can be and have been tested; their overall validity as concepts necessary for understanding group process has been confirmed. Individual testing, however, cannot proceed directly. Rather, the leader or participant-observer must entertain the interpretation as a hypothesis which, if true, will be revealed in other aspects of the individual's or the group's behavior. In this particular example, therefore, the teacher does not ask the student if he is challenging authority, but rather asks herself what else might be true if this interpretation is valid. The teacher in this case might notice other behaviors of this same student: e.g., he comes up frequently after class to disagree about particular points that have been made; he arrives late, especially on examination days; his manner is generally antagonistic; his work is a study in a casual-to-messy style. Notice that these additional behaviors are all consistent with the preliminary interpretations; they do not prove it to be correct, but add further weight to its confirmation. And likewise, they add further weight to the teacher's use of a concept such as hidden agenda to help deepen and enrich her understanding of the particular situation she is confronting. Within the context of the psychoanalytic model, to ignore or deny the role of unconscious processes would be comparable to ignoring the role of the autonomic nervous system in behavior.

Basic-Assumption Group Mode

W. R. Bion, an important contributor to our understanding of group process from an analytic perspective, examines the two types of agenda in his important distinction between what he terms a *work-group* mode and a *basic-assumption* mode (Bion, 1959; also see Thelen, 1959). When a group comes together to work, it has met to do something, to accomplish a task, to cooperate in order to get a job done. Members gear themselves to reality; they focus on rational ways to complete their task; to make the decisions necessary to solve the problems they encounter; to relate in a rational way to one another. A group functioning in this way is primarily concerned with its publicly stated agenda, with the more conscious level of functioning.

But, as Bion notes, if we were to focus our attention only on the work mode in analyzing group process, we would not only miss much of what takes place, but would also fail to understand some of the issues and problems that crop up and make working together difficult. Thus, it is also necessary to attend to the kinds of *unconscious basic assumptions* that characterize group process. It was Bion's contention that there are specific, recurrent unconscious themes and issues that are basic to all groups. We will examine these in more detail in our discussion of group development in Chapter 8. The unconscious emotional themes that describe the basic-assumption mode, however, involve such factors as hostility, flight or withdrawal, hope, helplessness, and dependency.

When group members glance furtively at one another while discussing the job they are doing, or when one member looks frequently at the group leader as though seeking approval, or when another member seems to reject almost automatically whatever the leader proposes, something is obviously taking place that cannot readily be understood solely in terms of the conscious task at hand. Bion suggests that concerns with leadership in particular—e.g., how to address the leader, how to handle the leader's style, what responses to make to the leader's suggestions—cannot be understood in conscious terms. Within the context of the basic-assumption mode, a group functions *as if* its members were following some shared, unconscious assumptions of why they have convened and what their purposes are. These basic assumptions are not tied into the realities at hand, nor are they designed to cope successfully with the group's tasks. Rather, they spring from deep emotional characteristics and needs within group members and tend to obstruct and divert the group from accomplishing its stated tasks.

A Critical Task. It would follow, therefore, that a critical task for a group to deal with in order to function more effectively involves understanding and working through its basic assumptions. The task or work agenda cannot be successfully negotiated until the hidden agenda is confronted and dealt with.

The point is simple but often overlooked by more rational conceptions of group process. In the psychoanalytic view, members' effectiveness in dealing with their tasks (i.e., the work of the group) can be thwarted by the unconscious basic assumptions of the group's hidden agenda. For example, some members may agree with the leader's directions more out of a need to be saved from feeling helpless and confused than because of the intrinsic merit of those suggestions for effectively handling the work issue that is faced. Or other members might resist good suggestions in an unconscious desire to rebel against all authority. In both cases, effective work is thwarted as members' unconscious relationships toward the leader interfere with their behaving rationally toward their tasks.

Decisions that a group makes that primarily serve such unconscious needs will crop up again and again; thus it is easy for a group to get bogged down and become unable to move effectively unless the group confronts its hidden agenda. Similarly, the leader may get agreement that is based more on members' unconscious needs than on the merits of his or her leadership and suggestions; or the leader may meet substantial resistance that has little to do with ideas and recommendations as such. Whichever the case may be, it should be apparent that these unconscious, basic assumptions can be destructive to effective behavior.

Member-to-Member Transferences

While much of Freud's, Bion's, and other psychoanalytic concepts of the group's unconscious life emphasize member relationships to the leader, it is important for us to recognize that a similar kind of unconscious transference can also be focused on member relationships with other members. Thus, the focus of unconscious basic assumptions is directed toward (1) the leader and (2) other members. The important unconscious themes that revolve around the leader involve members' relationships to authority, dependency, freedom, and individuality. The important themes that revolve around other members involve such issues as competition, assertiveness, intimacy, sexuality, envy, giving, sharing (Yalom, 1975). These too form part of the group's hidden agenda. They involve such factors as members' fears of competing against others and either winning or losing, or strong needs to win or lose (i.e., to fail). They may involve members' desires to be assertive or domineering. They may involve members' desires to become close and intimate with others, or fears of closeness and intimacy. They may involve members' envy of others in relation to approval of the leader, jealousies, inabilities to give and to share, and so forth.

Hidden agenda, then, provides a rich territory for exploring and understanding group process. The failure to deal with its implications and issues will inevitably cause a group to perform on a less than optimum level.

An Example

Nurse Riles has always been concerned with her femininity. She was brought up in a rather traditional way to believe that the proper role for a woman was to be relatively passive and nonassertive, especially in the presence of men. For her, being feminine is related to being nonassertive. In fact, whenever she begins to assert herself in a group she vaguely senses that she is behaving in an unfeminine manner. Consequently, she tends to altogether avoid asserting herself, or she stops short just as she begins to declare her own views within the group. Nurse Riles, however, is also very frustrated and angry—especially at herself. She feels she has some good ideas to contribute. But her habitual passivity and silence makes her consent to letting others take the lead and have their ideas accepted, even when she believes that her own views may be as good and often better. Her smiling and agreeable presence is noted at group meetings; yet her underlying anger and conflict are more effective determinants of her actions. Although she may outwardly approve of the ideas that lead to a group decision, she frequently drags her feet when it is time for the final decisions to be determined. Often she is a puzzle to others in her group; they think that she is agreeing with their suggestions and yet wonder why she doesn't pitch in eagerly in following them.

In this example, we have a member's own hidden agenda, involving a link between assertiveness and femininity. This hidden agenda profoundly influences Nurse Riles' behavior within the group, and has a very detrimental effect on the whole group and its ability to function as a unit. Decisions are made and seemingly accepted, and yet are not carried out very well. Assertiveness, in this case, takes the form of an *implicit* refusal to carry out group decisions; this is covered over by what appears to be *explicit* acceptance of such decisions. That is, Nurse Riles does assert herself, but in a concealed way by her slow or grudging implementation of decisions. Clearly, a group with such members cannot hope to function well until these hidden agendas are brought to the surface so they can be dealt with; that is, until assertiveness is part of the group's explicit mode of working together.

A Summary. We have learned that all groups, no matter what their purposes may be, partake of two rather different kinds of process. The one is relatively conscious and rational and is concerned with the group's stated task agenda. This is the activity we tend to see when we observe a group in action. For example, we see the group's leader make a suggestion and members comment on it; we see decisions being made and members contributing variously to making those decisions; we see problems being discussed and solutions sought. The other process is less conscious and less rational; it reflects a set of basic assumptions under which members operate but of which they and we as casual observers tend to be unaware. More careful observation, however, may reveal that some members act as though they were angry with the leader for reasons far removed from the task at hand, or are pleased with someone else in the group—again, for reasons not immediately understandable in terms of that person's contributions to the task. Members seem to act as though guided by some basic assumptions that are less rational and more concerned with underlying emotions than those involved with their task.

We can expect hidden agendas to develop within all groups and to be focused on leadership and on other members. That is, both leaders and other members serve as targets for the playing out of unconscious feelings and concerns. Typically, leaders are the focus of members' concerns wth authority, freedom, and dependency; members are the focus of concerns with competition, intimacy, sharing, and such.

Work groups are always affected by basic-assumption behaviors; thus to understand and to intervene effectively in group process, we must be aware of a group's unconscious level of behavior as well as the surface manifestations of work-group activity. This is a critical point. It is not possible either to understand or effectively work with a group unless unconscious basic assumptions—the group's hidden agenda—are dealt with as they relate to conscious work and task activity.

For example, if a group's resistance to adopting a leader's suggestions is based more on unconscious than conscious reasons, no matter how hard that leader tries to rationally persuade members of the reasonableness of her suggestions, she will fail to convince. She will have invested her efforts inappropriately if she focuses on rational persuasion for issues that have an unconscious nonrational basis.

Why Hidden Agendas?

There are several reasons why all groups can be expected to develop some types of hidden agenda in addition to their publicly stated work agendas. We will briefly examine three of these reasons: unresolved feelings, learned habits of public behavior, and fears of vulnerability.

Unresolved Feelings.　Most of the examples and the discussion of hidden agendas up to this point have emphasized their basis in unresolved unconscious feelings and conflicts: e.g., Nurse Riles' concern that assertiveness is not feminine. All of us arrive at our ongoing group and social settings with a variety of still unresolved issues from our past. Stock, Whitman, and Lieberman (1958) referred to these as the individual's *nuclear conflict.* They involve any number of past hurts and deprivations that remain as scars and tender places liable to be opened up again in the right situation.

Stock and her associates offer the example of a man from a large family who as a child continually tried to win the attention of his parents, to separate himself from his siblings and to appear as someone unique and worthy of their special attention. This demand for recognition has become the adult's unresolved nuclear conflict. When this man is within a group situation, he unconsciously feels in the same competitive circumstances again—the other group members are in a sense his siblings and the leader, his parents. So he begins to strive anew for recognition and special attention; this time, however, he seeks it from the group's leader.

In other words, the group has become a setting that serves to trigger this man's unresolved conflicts; it becomes a stage upon which he plays out these unresolved underlying issues. In one way or another, we all play our such issues in our ongoing group behavior. Such nuclear issues are at the base of a group's complex constellation of hidden agendas.

Habits of Public Behavior.　As we all grow up within a particular culture, we learn certain ways to publicly express our feelings and our ideas; that is, we learn certain habits of public expression. For example, some people have learned that it is not appropriate to express feelings; others have learned that feelings are something to be expressed and shared with others. Within our culture there are many, including those who enter the health professions, who believe that it is not appropriate to express or share their feelings in public (see Buck et al., 1974; Learmonth et al., 1959). Such people have learned to be somewhat reserved—to maintain at least a facade of calm and cool rationality.

Such behavior represents learned habits of public expression and not necessarily a manifestation of actual feelings. When individuals experience emotions but submerge them, those feelings tend to gain an indirect expression. They are thus not directly observable, but become part of the private background behavior that is influential even though "hidden." For example, Nurse Riles may have learned that she should not publicly express the anger that she feels when she fails to assert herself; but that anger does exist and is expressed indirectly in the form of reluctant, grudging compliance with decisions that are made.

Indirect expressions of feelings (or even ideas) comprise a rich source of material for a group's hidden agenda, and as such can serve to confuse and to thwart effective group communication and functioning until they are more directly confronted and dealt with.

Fears of Vulnerability. A third, related basis for the development of hidden agendas involves the fears we all have of being vulnerable. To be direct in saying what we believe or feel, for example, can open us to the possibility of attack from others. So we may choose to be indirect or to withhold in order to protect ourselves. And yet, as we have already noted, while we do so, we become contributors to the developing hidden agenda of those groups and relationships in which we are involved.

Rational Conflicts

Not all conflicts and disagreements within groups are based on unconscious assumptions. There are many clear and definitely rational bases for disagreements; these, however, can usually be confronted directly and dealt with in a relatively reasonable manner; sensible compromises can be achieved. However, when the basis for conflict (or even for inappropriate agreement—e.g., saying "yes" to a foolish proposal) is more deeply rooted, then rational solutions are hard to achieve. Problems may recur and never be resolved; compromises may be tentative, and acceptance of leadership and of group decisions weak.

SYMBOLIZATION

Before we leave our consideration of the unconscious aspects of group process (we return to them again in Chapter 8), it will be helpful to consider briefly what can be termed the *symbolization process* (also see Mills 1964). Nowhere are unconscious dynamics revealed more than in the symbolization of issues. A few examples will illustrate this.

The group is together for its first meeting for a treatment review of Mr. R. Although several members know one another from past contacts, most are only passing acquaintances and several are new to the group. The leader, Dr. Winch, initiates the discussion about Mr. R. An intern comments on the difficulties in dealing with Mr. R. because of a language barrier. A nurse suggests that even without this barrier it would be difficult because Mr. R. speaks so softly that he is difficult to hear. Additional comments are made, all focusing on issues of communication and understanding of the patient, Mr. R.

In this example, the patient has difficulty in speaking English; he also speaks softly and people must ask him to repeat what he says. There is little doubt that one aspect of the case involves matters of communication and understanding. Yet in view of the group's interaction it appears that something more may be involved. In particular, perhaps the intensive focus on issues of communication and understanding also symbolizes or represents an underlying issue for the group. Are these doctors and nurses also introducing, via the patient's problems of communication, their own group's issues involving understanding and communication?

This appears to be a reasonable hypothesis, one that a careful analyst of group process might wish to make and to examine further. It is not surprising, of course, that persons who meet together for the first time possibly have problems in communication and understanding. This is the very type of issue that an effective group leader should look for in trying to help the group work together more effectively.

A group of students, all taking a course in group process, began to focus the discussion on the members' other courses. Karen noted that she used to be afraid to speak out in class until she realized that others in her classes were just as frightened. Walt mentioned that he used to think that he must be a stupid person compared to others; and yet when he compared his grades with theirs he realized that they were having the same kinds of difficulties. Marianne recalled a man in one of her classes who had always arrived carrying a briefcase; his appearance of purpose and intelligence had made her feel intimidated, small, and stupid by comparison. Later she learned that he was getting a C in the course, while she was a B student.

In this discussion, no member of the group made direct reference to the group that was now meeting and holding this discussion. The entire discussion was focused on the students' experiences in other classes and how they had learned from those experiences that everyone was "in the same boat together." In a sense their conversation was reflecting similar doubts about their present group. Perhaps they were also saying, in essence: "I don't really know much about group process and I am frightened and unsure of myself. But maybe no one in this room knows much about group process; we are all equal in our ignorance, so perhaps I shouldn't be so frightened and unsure of myself." In other words, the reference to things outside their own group symbolized or represented issues that were simultaneously "internal" to their group and to the members' ongoing experiences.

Hypothesis, Not Fact. It is important to realize that the statement that the ongoing conversation in this example symbolizes or represents an issue to the group itself is really a hunch or a hypothesis. As a hypothesis, it must both be seriously considered and tested. That is, the leader-observer must be able to formulate such hypotheses from the material of ongoing group discussion and be able to test them for their validity. But direct testing (e.g., by asking group members if they are really also talking about themselves) will not invariably confirm a correct hypothesis about symbolized, unconscious matters. In fact, there is often resistance to such interpretations.

The leader, therefore, may entertain the hypothesis but not immediately share it, deciding to wait until more material surfaces. For example, a member may eventually hint at the possibility that the members are really also talking about themselves and their own issues with one another. Or the leader may decide that it is best to intervene as though his or her interpretive hypothesis were correct. In this case the leader would assume that members are worried about their knowledge and are unsure of themselves and would thus benefit from some supportive comments from him or her. Or the leader might assume that members are having some difficulty in communicating with one another and decide to actively clarify what is being said.

Sources for Symbolization

Authority and peer relations are considered two critical areas of unconscious work within groups, and as such provide a rich source of material for frequent symbolization. We would expect groups to have discussions about problems that seem to be external to themselves (e.g., talking about Mr. R.'s communication problems) that involve issues of authority, dependency, control, freedom, and independence on the one hand, or of intimacy, friendship, acceptance, and rejection, on the other. These give us a useful clue as to what issues are very likely internal to the group as well.

A student group that is about to end, for example, may talk at great length about the trouble that its patients are having with leaving the hospital after a lengthy illness. They go on and on about the patients' need for the hospital and its support, the patients' difficulties in making the break and going home again, and so forth. The hypothesis is that the group members may not only be talking about the patients' difficulties but their own difficulties in terminating their group and in leaving the friendships and support they have in the group. We might test this hypothesis by directly asking such a question as: "Is termination of our own group something that we should talk about here?" or by assuming its validity and acting upon it—e.g., "I have some feelings about our own group's ending and would like to talk about these."

SUMMARY AND CONCLUSIONS

The theoretical position presented in this chapter is that unconscious themes and issues pervade all groups. Typically, these divert energy and attention away from using a group's resources most effectively to get its various tasks accomplished. These themes especially center around leadership and authority on the one hand and on member-to-member relations on the other. Individuals bring to their group interactions a background of ways of relating to leaders and peers; many of these distort a productive mode of functioning and thereby prove troublesome for the group. Often, these unconscious themes and issues can be ascertained through an examination of the symbolic meaning of the surface issues that capture the group's attention. Skillful leaders or even members soon learn to listen with their third ear, to hear what else is meant by what is being said and to understand what is meant by the things that are left unsaid.

6

Symbolic Interactionism: Meaning and Identity in Group Behavior

According to the psychoanalytic perspective, what has survived from people's unconscious past affects a goodly portion of the behavior that can be observed in groups. By contrast, according to the *symbolic interactionist view*, the immediate here-and-now ongoing situation is more critical in observing and understanding group process. This theory derives from the writings of G. H. Mead (1934): it owes much to the analyses later proposed by Blumer (1966) and by Strauss (1969), among others. Although it goes by many other names, some aspects of the thinking of Goffman (1959; 1974) and of Garfinkel (1967) are similar as well.

There are several key ideas embodied in the theory. While they appear to be simple, they are actually rather powerful in their implications for our analysis and understanding of group process. We will consider seven basic points.

MEANINGS GUIDE BEHAVIOR

People behave in terms of the meanings of acts and objects. In this view, our behavior is not the outcome of unthinking reflexes such as an automatic knee jerk; rather, our behavior results from the meanings and the understandings we have about our own and about others' behavior. For example, a flashing light is not simply a stimulus that sends impulses from our receptors through our brain centers to our muscles leading to action. The flashing light comes to have meaning (e.g., a warning signal of an approaching train), and our behavior is in response to this meaning. In similar fashion, the behavior of another member of a group is not simply a meaningless stimulus that automatically produces a response in us; our response develops on the basis of the meanings we attach to that person's behavior and the understandings we have about it.

Meaning mediates our behavior; it stands between the stimulus and our response. This suggests that the analyst must pay careful attention to the ways in which people attribute meaning to their own and to others' behaviors. We are especially concerned with the ways in which groups develop the meanings for members' behavior that are special to that group. For example, arriving late to a meeting, like the flashing light, by itself is an act without meaning until a group confers its own special meaning on that act. Our interest is in the ways in which these meanings develop and the behavioral consequences that follow. The act of arriving late may mean any number of things: e.g., "I am of sufficiently high status in this group that I can arrive late without penalty"; "I am arriving late because I am angry with this group"; "I am arriving late because there are priorities in my life that are higher than coming on time to this meeting." How people will behave toward the latecomer will be a function of the meanings they attribute to this behavior.

MEANINGS EMERGE IN INTERACTION

Meanings, so important to our behavior, are not intrinsic to acts or to objects, bur rather emerge in the course of group interaction. The act of arriving late, as we noted, has no intrinsic meaning; its meaning emerges within the particular social context of the group in which it occurs and in which it evokes a particular response.

Let us take another example, the object we call a chair. If the meaning of that object were intrinsic to it, then "chair" would always have the same meaning regardless of the setting or the circumstances of its use. However, a chair may be used to sit upon, as firewood, as a ladder, as a weapon to throw at someone, as a defensive shield (e.g., the lion tamer's chair), and so forth. The meaning, then, does not reside in the object as such but emerges as a function of how the object is used. Admittedly, we are rarely concerned with the meaning of chairs. We are more interested in the behavior of persons in group interaction. The same principle is said to hold. The meaning that attaches to another person's behavior emerges in our interaction with that person.

In other words, meaning does not exist prior to or separate from our encounter with others; it emerges as we and they interact together, just as the meaning of that chair develops and changes as its use changes. Late arrival means something different depending on the circumstances of its occurrence, including who arrives late, to what they arrive late, and so forth. Thus, the meaning does not lie within the act or object; it is not intrinsic to the behavior of arriving late; its meaning emerges within a social context. The meaning of acts (e.g., arriving late) and objects (e.g., chairs) is conferred by and through social interaction.

MEANINGS DEPEND ON OTHERS

An important implication of the second point is that the meanings of acts, objects, and behaviors, being embedded in and emerging from social interaction, depend upon more than one person for their realization. Several illustrative examples will help us better understand this important point. Sullivan (1953) offers the example of a baby that is crying and a mother who responds by picking up and comforting the baby. The point is that the act of crying does not contain any intrinsic meaning but rather serves to *evoke* meaning. It is the mother's response to the infant's crying that confers meaning upon the act itself: i.e., crying comes to mean "receiving comfort." In this example, meaning emerges from the infant's behavior *and* the mother's response; thus the meaning is lodged or located in their social interaction and not in the act itself.

Let us take a second example, the case of the borrower and the lender (from Dewey & Bentley, 1949). The meaning of being a borrower is dependent on there being another person, the lender; in turn, the meaning of lender requires that there be a borrower. To be a borrower, in other words, requires that someone else be a lender, and vice versa. The meaning of one depends on the acts of the other. The two persons mutually create the meaning that each party comes to have. In this example, the meanings involve their actual identities: i.e., one has the identity of a borrower and the other that of a lender. Their identities do not exist in isolation nor as properties of the individuals as such. The meaning emerges as they interact and play out their parts together.

We will soon follow up this point. For now, however, it is important to notice that the meaning of a person's identity—that is, who one is—is socially defined and socially located. Who we are therefore is in an important sense not something that is intrinsic to us, but rather is something that emerges within social interaction. This is true not only for borrowers and lenders, but also for all kinds of identities, including professional identities as doctors, nurses, social workers, psychiatrists, and so forth. In each social encounter, therefore, we create our identity; its meaning is a function not only of our behavior but also of others' responses. Together we create the meaning of our identity. The student of group process is witness to and participant in interactions in which meanings and identities are being created.

The Act and Its Completion.   The symbolic interactionist theory offers us a detailed specification of this third important point by noting that the gestures of one person are the preliminary, tentative beginnings of what will become a complete social act (i.e., an interaction or transaction). The act is completed and its meaning emerges as other people respond to these beginning gestures. For example, John is angry and so raises his arm, extends it, makes a fist, and swings it back and forth in a jabbing motion toward his physiotherapist; it is the latter's response to the gesture that completes the act and gives it the meaning it will have. Thus, as the physiotherapist smiles and pushes John's arm aside, saying, "Great energy, now get going on your exercises," we see this as a gesture that does not mean anger. If the response were to be a frightened attempt to get out of the way of what was felt to be an aggressive punch, then the meaning that would emerge is something very different.

The critical point is that meanings emerge in social interaction as a function of how the parties to that interaction behave and respond to one another. The meanings do not exist as anything but tentative proposals until others respond and complete the proposal, thereby endowing it with meaning. This brings us to the related fourth point.

CHARACTERISTICS ARE SOCIALLY CREATED

In the symbolic interactionist view, others play an important role in confirming or in denying the meanings we tentatively propose through our gestures. Gestures in this context include the language we use, our appearance, and our mannerisms, as well as the settings within which we behave. If others respond to our gestures so as to confirm their provisional meanings, then the meaning we initiate is completed. For example, if we raise our fist in anger and others respond appropriately to confirm that meaning, then indeed, the meaning of our raised fist is as we intended. However, as in the example of John and his physiotherapist, others may respond in ways that deny the preliminary meanings we initiated; they may laugh at our raised fist and thereby confer a different meaning upon the act. Remember, it is the response of others that completes our actions and thereby confirms or denies their meaning. In this sense, therefore, meanings clearly arise in social interaction and are not truly present prior to or separate from that interaction.

This is an important point. It suggests that characteristics we may take to be an aspect of the individual are better understood as aspects of social interaction involving that individual and others. These others serve their part in confirming or in refuting the characteristics in question. Since we may be one of those others, our own actions can serve to confirm or to deny meanings. We are always thereby bound up in others' lives. Let us take some helpful examples based on typical group interaction.

> One member of the group seems to lack initiative; he always waits for others to take the lead and to get things going. Our response is to ignore him, let him remain silent, and to take on the initiative ourselves.

> In another group, one member always seems to be the scapegoat, the butt of everyone's jokes or anger. Whatever group she enters, people automatically give her this scapegoat identity. People resent any efforts she makes to change from being the scapegoat.

> A group of recent cardiac patients contains one man who complains that since his attack he feels that there is little reason for him to go on living; he can't do any of the activities he used to do, especially around the house, where he has become almost a helpless invalid because everyone does everything for him.

In each of these examples, we have one person who seems to possess a particular characteristic or a consistent way of behaving: a passive man without initiative; a scapegoat; a helpless invalid. It is easy for us to attribute this characteristic to something within the person. So we come to think of the man as "being" passive, as lacking any initiative, perhaps even as being a bit ignorant or uncaring. We think of the scapegoat as having "the kind of personality" that grates on others' nerves, as someone who deserves to be ridiculed and joked about. We think of the cardiac patient as being a helpless invalid, as one who has no contribution to make and so must be totally cared for. According to the symbolic interactionist model, what we have failed to consider in each case are the ways in which the person's behavior has its meaning confirmed through the actions of others, how others' responses establish the person's characteristics.

Remember, it is the responses of others that complete the social act initiated by the person's gestures and which thereby render it meaningful. Thus the man in the first example does not have the passive qualities independent of the way others treat him. If his behavior lacks initiative and he seems to be passive, we must examine the ways in which the responses of others help confer this meaning. Indeed, other people's response of ignoring him and taking on the initiative themselves clearly helps to sustain his identity as one without initiative. Likewise, the cardiac patient is not a helpless invalid nor the woman a scapegoat without others in the setting (e.g., the family, the group) to confirm these characteristics.

IDENTITY HAS A SOCIALLY LOCATED MEANING

One of the key concepts in the symbolic interactionist model of group process is the concept of *identity*. Basically, identity refers to an individual's sense of who he or she is, their concept of themselves as a social object or social being. Identity locates people in a social world of others. It involves roles, the things people do that place them within a social network. For example, job roles help give people an identity within a society or within an organization. Roles within a family likewise give people an identity, a place and location within the family as a group. But identity includes more than roles; it also involves appearance, gestures, and mannerisms that help locate the individual as a particular kind of person. Thus, people may behave aggressively or sympathetically, they may be cold or empathetic, they may be passive or active, and so forth. These are all qualities of character that also help locate individuals within a social space, within the social world human beings pass through in their everyday lives.

Identity—basically, who we are—is felt to be one of the most critical qualities we have. Identity helps organize our experiences, staves off anxiety, defines a sense of meaning and purpose; our identity helps provide a sense of continuity and stability to our lives. A confusion of identity or an excessively diffused identity can leave us vulnerable and disturbed. Adolescence is an especially critical period in the formation of identity. It is a period marked by the search for an identity—a location and set of characteristics for defining who we are. It is often a period of difficulty and tension as the individual tries on different identities, becoming various kinds of persons while searching for the one on which he or she will finally focus and to which some commitment will be made.

A person's identity can be seen as a hard-won achievement, as something that is both accomplished and continually worked at so that it will be maintained. One's identity is never fully settled or completed; it is always in the process of evolving. The maintenance of identity is a critical issue that is implicated in all social and interpersonal relations. This occurs primarily because our identity, the very person we are, is not simply something we carry about within us, but rather, as with all other matters we have been considering, it *gains* its meaning and hence *maintains* its meaning as an outcome of social interaction. In other words, our identity is accomplished, established, and maintained in and through the acts of others. Therefore, who we are is significantly influenced by the ways in which others respond to us. It is their response to our preliminary gestures and indications of our identity that either confirms us as having that identity or refutes us and forces a crisis of identity.

> John L., age 20, has a spinal cord injury. His initial response to his paralysis was to become totally dependent and a true invalid. His mother, overcome by grief, responded by "overmothering" him; thus he became further involved in identifying himself as a hopelessly bedridden invalid. The hospital staff began to respond to this dependent identity in a very different way. He was not brought everything he cried out for; he was made to "do it himself," "get it for himself." The staff began to respond to him as a young man who could do many things for himself; he could move himself about, even get a job. In time, be began to see himself differently; he began to take on a new identity as a result of the staff's manner of treating him.

This example suggests two related points. First, identity is a critical concept that is implicated in all social interaction. Knowing this can help us better understand what happens as persons come together in groups to ineract. Much of what goes on involves a negotiation over and about identities; group interaction can be viewed as involving the confirmation or denial of members' identities. (We will shortly further

examine this process of negotiation.) Second, identity is not a posses-
sion of the individual as such, but rather gains its meaning, as do all
objects and acts, by the ways in which others respond. Thus, who we
are, our identity, has a socially located meaning. Our identity is embedded in the group process. We accomplish it by virtue of the groups in
which we are socialized; and we maintain that identity by virtue of locating ourselves in groups that respond to us in ways that confirm that
identity.

Let us take another simple but informative example to illustrate
what we mean. We will look at a small instance of behavior between a
nurse and a patient, in which the content of the interaction as well as
its style clearly conveys the identities of the two parties. The nurse
makes gestures that indicate, "My identity is that of a nurse", the patient responds in ways that confirm that identity for the nurse while
making gestures that indicate, "I am the patient" and receiving confirmation for that identity.

> NURSE: Please step into that room and use this small bottle to give
> me a urine sample; then when you have finished bring it out
> here and leave it on this table. Then go into that other room and
> remove all your clothing, including your socks and shorts.
> MALE PATIENT: O.K. (he leaves to carry out her orders)

We need not belabor the point. In this example we have the identities of each confirmed by the actions of the other. The patient's acceptance of the requests (or orders) informs about the identity of the
person making the request. If the janitor had given the same requests,
he would hardly have gotten similar compliance. The patient's compliance helps confirm this as a medical setting in which the other person,
behaving in a properly authoritative manner, can make requests that
bear compliance; but these requests would be highly unusual and worthy of rejection if they occurred in another context. Further, if these
two were to meet at a party and if the nurse made the same requests,
it would undoubtedly be taken as a joke and not something that confirmed her as a nurse and him as a patient.

This fifth point in our consideration of the symbolic interactionist
approach suggests that we can understand much about group process
if we think about people's behaviors as attempts to establish and maintain identities, to negotiate over identities, to confirm, or deny identities to one another. It is necessary to view social interaction within

groups in these terms to uncover the myriad ways in which people engage in the identity maintaining-confirming-denying process as they interact together. This then brings us to a sixth, related point.

IDENTITY IS RECRUITED

Up to this point, it may appear as though a person's identity is a very fragile thing. It is critical to well being and yet seems totally beyond control because its meaning derives from the ways in which others respond to the individual. This is far from the actual truth, however. Persons actively recruit the responses they need from others so that they can be the kind of person they are. Three important concepts are relevant at this point: *selectivity, self-presentation,* and *alter-casting* (see Sampson, 1976).

Selectivity. One way in which persons achieve and maintain an identity in a relatively stable state involves selectivity both about the others with whom they interact and about the kinds of topics and issues on which they ineract. Birds of a feather do generally flock together. People with similar perspectives and ideas tend to associate together more than people with widely differing points of view. In this way, they are more likely to be confirmed than denied in their identities. We can learn much about another person, thereby, by noting the kinds of groups with which he or she tends to become involved.

But there is more than selectivity of interaction partners that is involved. Everyone must associate with others whose behavior might challenge and threaten their identities. We tend to handle this by being highly selective in the kinds of material that we are willing to discuss; we choose material that is hospitable to our existing identities. Or we may respond by anger, rejection, or even withdrawal should potentially threatening topics emerge within a group's discussion. In this way, we take a very active part in protecting and in maintaining our identity; we seek persons and topics that are likely to confirm rather than to deny the identity we have.

A person, for example, may refuse to talk about sexual matters or may respond with indignation or anger when such topics are brought up. While there are many reasons for this behavior, one that should not be overlooked is the role which the behavior of not appearing to be sexually interested plays in their identity. They protect their identity as "one who is nonsexual" by refusing to participate even in discussions that deal with sexual topics. In other words, their identity ("nonsexual being") is maintained by a selectivity of participation.

Another kind of selectivity also operates to help people take an active part in maintaining their identities. This involves a process of *selective attention*. We may frequently interact with persons who could challenge our sense of who we are; yet, in defense of our identity, we become highly selective in what we attend to and what we remember about those interactions. We can become inattentive to material that would threaten our accepted ways; we can become selective in what we remember of our encounters. Accurate perception of others' responses to us can often be sufficiently threatening to our identities that we are motivated not to see clearly, not to hear well, and not to remember accurately. The degree and nature of the selective distortions in communication and understanding that occur within a group are truly amazing. The student of group process can learn much about what is important to group members by noting the kinds of selective inattentions that occur.

> Nurse Kelley seems oblivious to feedback; in particular, she seems to ignore all efforts to dissuade her from doing what she feels is supposed to be done. She appears to be unable to hear disagreements with her own opinions; even when someone points out to her that someone has just offered a suggestion that disagrees with hers, she disposes of this by nodding affirmatively and then proceeding as though no disagreement were heard. Continued observation of this selectivity bears out the impression that "being right," "being in charge", "being dominant," are all critical aspects of Nurse Kelley's identity; that is, the maintenance of her identity requires that she be right all the time. So, when she gets herself into a situation with people who disagree with her, she handles this by selectively not attending to what would otherwise deny her identity as someone who is "always right."

Self-Presentation. Beyond selectivity, however, there are other ways of actively recruiting support and confirmation for our identities. Goffman (1959) introduced the concept of *impression management*, which posits that all persons employ some kinds of self-presentations so as to manage the impressions that others form of them. The ways in which we present ourselves to others, the manner of our appearance, our style of talk, our vocabulary, the clothing we wear, the props we employ, the ways in which we manage the settings—all these are indicative of the attempt to gain confirmation of our identity. The point is a simple one. If identity gains its meaning by virtue of the responses that others make to an individual's gestures, then, in knowledge of this, that individual attempts to manage those responses by making proper gestures: i.e., gestures that will evoke the kinds of responses that are needed to confirm a particular identity.

In a sense, we are like actors on a stage, engaged in a performance designed to create and sustain a character by using our audience in appropriate ways. If a woman dresses and acts seductively, she should not be surprised if others respond to her as a sex object and thereby confirm what at some level (perhaps deeply unconscious) she sees or wishes herself to be. If a man speaks in formal ways, selects a vocabulary that tends to be highly technical and sophisticated, dresses in conservative and formal clothing even in more casual settings, again, he is managing others' responses to him: he is actively involved in recruiting a set of responses from others that will define him and give him a desired identity. Thus, the analyst of group process must attend carefully to the ways people present themselves and attempt to manage the impression that others have of them; from this we can learn much about people's identities and much therefore about the ways in which they interact in groups.

Alter-Casting. If self-presentation involves managing others' responses to us by doing something to our own behavior and appearance, alter-casting is a technique by which we try to do something directly to others. Specifically, we cast these others (others = alter) into relationships which, if they accept them, will place us in the desired reciprocal relationship that offers us the identity we desire. Suppose, for example, that a woman of 45 whose children are now nearly grown and about to leave the nest really cannot tolerate the sense of herself as anything but a young mother of still-young children. One way of attempting to sustain this identity is to continue to cast her children into the roles of little children. She may do this by the way she talks to them ("You will always be my little baby"), the way she treats them ("Here, let me help you with that"), and so forth. To the extent that her children accept their roles as little kids, she will maintain herself in the reciprocal role and identity of a still-young mother.

Most of us engage in alter-casting when we seek another's advice on some pressing matter. Alice says, "Jane, as my friend, I wonder if you could tell me what you think I should do." Alice has cast Jane into the role "friend" so that she may be responded to in the reciprocal role of "friend" and receive a friend's advice rather than something more objective that she may not wish to hear. Alice clues Jane in, in other words, to the kind of response she is willing to hear.

IDENTITY CONFIRMATION IS LARGELY OUTSIDE AWARENESS

We come now to the final point involving the symbolic interactionist perspective: that our identity confirmation and maintenance is largely outside our awareness. None of what we have said about this model should necessarily imply that people act with full conscious awareness or intentionality regarding the processes of establishing and maintaining their identities. The language we use—for example, speaking about managing an impression, selecting persons and topics for conversation, casting others into roles, etc.—admittedly may imply a conscious, even willfully manipulative actor. Indeed, while some persons may engage in these processes of identity maintenance in a conscious way, it is more usual to discover that these are processes we all engage in without much awareness or sensitivity to what we are doing or even why. In fact, we may resist another's suggestion that we may be setting the stage for evoking responses from others and for sustaining a particular identity. The analyst's language makes the process seem more conscious than it is.

NEGOTIATING REALITY

Before concluding the consideration of the symbolic interactionist approach to group process, we need to examine some of its applications and implications for practice in the health professions. Two examples will be briefly examined: arriving at a medical diagnosis and the dying patient. But first we need to focus our attention on the idea that reality (e.g., meanings and identities) is negotiated in social interaction.

The symbolic interactionist position is very clear on this point about reality. Basically, the social world is not seen to be an objective realm of facts to be apprehended and known through simple observation. Rather, the social world is created by persons who interact and interpret it. This is the essential message contained in the points just considered. Meaning is not intrinsic to objects or persons, but rather develops and emerges from the ways in which persons interact and interpret their world. Who we are, as we have already noted, is something that is created by and through social interaction.

What this means, therefore, is that social reality is something over which persons have some say. They are not grasping a reality that exists independently of their efforts to grasp it. Rather, in the acts of trying to know reality, they *create* a reality. Naturally individuals may attempt to know the world in different ways; therefore, a process of negotiation usually takes place. That is, people will attempt to negotiate the nature of their social world, trying to get their version or their interpretation accepted by others. These others, in turn, are trying to get their version accepted as well. The social reality that emerges, therefore, is the outcome of a negotiation process.

Medical Diagnosis

In a medical assessment, according to the symbolic interactionist view, the actual process of interviewing or interrogating is not seen simply to involve a procedure for obtaining information about the nature of the patient's medical reality; rather, it is seen as a procedure that joins health professional with patient in establishing or creating the patient's medical reality.

The medical psychoanalyst, Balint (1957; also see Scheff, 1968), provides us with a useful way of understanding the negotiation process that occurs in medical diagnosis. Balint spent several years meeting with physicians and discussing their practice with them. His ideas, therefore, are based on his understanding of how these physicians engaged in their practice. Balint referred to the process of medical diagnosis as involving *offers* and *responses*. Suppose the physician sees patients early in their illness, before there is a clear diagnosis. At that point, we may note

> that the patients, so to speak, offer or propose various illnesses, and that they have to go on offering new illnesses until between doctor and patient an agreement can be reached resulting in the acceptance by both of them of one of the illnesses as justified. (p. 18)

In other words, the doctor and patient negotiate over the diagnosis: i.e., over the nature of social reality. The patient makes offers of possibilities for an illness or reasons why medical attention is needed; the doctor, in turn, responds to these offers and makes counter-offers. Finally, some kind of negotiated compromise is reached.

Balint further notes the role of what he terms the physician's "apostolic function" in this negotiation process. The apostolic function involves the health professional's often vague but important sense of how a patient should behave when ill. His or her mission is to help patients see this proper pattern of behavior and accept its legitimacy. In negotiating over diagnoses, therefore, the doctor fulfills the apostolic function by trying to get the patient to accept the kind of illness that the doctor feels is proper: i.e., to become a good patient and not a problem patient. Typically, the good patient is one who has a treatable illness. Much negotiation thereby involves the health professional's efforts to help the patient accomplish a treatable illness.

By referring to medical diagnoses as involving a negotiation over the nature and the meaning of reality, we are using the symbolic interactionist model to emphasize the process by which reality—in this case, the reality of a medical diagnosis—is accomplished via the interactions between doctor and patient. Of course, the negotiation does not simply involve doctor and patient; it is implicated whenever the patient and any health professional meet to evaluate the patient's status. Each of these encounters can be seen as a part of a negotiation process.

Much the same kind of negotiations can be seen within group process as well. In this case, members are negotiating about the nature of their social reality together: e.g., who each member is, what their functions are, why they have convened, what their legitimate purposes are, how they will know if they have reached their goals, and so on. The interactions among members, in this view, take on a new light. We see them likewise making offers and receiving responses and counter-offers. We see the group as attempting to achieve a negotiated settlement about its joint social reality.

The Dying Patient

Glaser and Strauss (1964) offer us a useful concept, the *closed-awareness context*, for examining the dying patient in the hospital. An awareness context involves the degree to which the several parties involved in an interaction know the identity of self and other. In an open context, all parties are aware of who the others are; in a closed-awareness context, one of the parties does not know the identity of the others. For example, a male homosexual in a group may keep his homosexual identity a secret from the other members. The awareness context is closed in that they do not know one important aspect of his identity.

A closed-awareness context in the case of the dying patient exists whenever the staff of nurses and physicians know that the patient is dying but try to keep this "identity" unknown to the patient. Thus they act as though the patient is going to recover and have a long future life, while knowing that the patient faces imminent death. In this example, the efforts of the hospital staff are directed toward *avoiding* negotiating with the patient over the identity as one who is dying. That is, they do not wish to negotiate, but to keep things secret.

Glaser and Strauss outline some important consequences that follow from these efforts to keep the awareness context closed from patient's knowledge and possible negotiation: (1) The staff acts as though everything were normal, at least when in sight or hearing of the patient. They speak of the future, of when the patient gets out, and so forth. However, because of the strain that is involved in keeping the patient in the dark regarding the pending death, the staff tends to avoid close contacts with the dying patient. They physically separate themselves from the patient, thereby helping to ensure that the identity (as one who is dying) will not leak out. (2) There are dangers to such collusion among staff members; great teamwork and implicit understanding are required to keep the secret and to prevent the patient from suspecting what everyone else knows. The day and night staff, however, never get to practice together and so may provide the patient with contradictory pieces of information that increase suspicion. This adds further strain to the staff relations with the patient as well as to relations among staff members: e.g., getting angry or upset with a staff member who leaks too much information to the patient. (3) Much of the burden for the patients day-by-day care falls to the nursing staff. The strain on them is greater than on the physicians, who may visit only briefly with the patient and thus who need not portray their parts for any sustained period of time.

While there are other consequences, the preceding example provides a good sense of what happens when the negotiation over reality systematically attempts to exclude one party from the process. In this case, the effort is made to exclude the patient from the defining process by withholding the very information that he or she would need in order to participate in it.

We need not focus entirely on the dying patient in order to see aspects of this same process at work in other contexts of relevance to the health professional. The group member who has a secret identity (e.g., the homosexual), or the member who has an identity that others are trying to keep from them (e.g., members implicitly cooperating to maintain a member as a scapegoat but never explicitly facing up to what they are doing) are other examples in which this model can be useful.

SUMMARY AND CONCLUSIONS

The essential feature of the symbolic interactionist analysis of group process is its emphasis on the role that ongoing interaction plays in creating social reality: i.e., in creating meanings and identities. To use this model, it is necessary to examine the here-and-now interaction between persons and to see that interaction as providing identities to the participants. Thus, it is vital to pay attention to one's role as a participant in the process whereby identities are being formed.

In a sense, there is no such thing as pure observation; people actively influence what they are observing. Our presence and reactions to others play a critical role in influencing the identity they come to have. This critical role is highlighted especially in the examination of the ways in which reality is negotiated. For example, the very process of interviewing or interrogating a patient in order to make an assessment and diagnosis is not simply a neutral fact-finding venture; it embodies a process of negotiation in which we and they (and other health professionals) attempt to negotiate a meaning to the patient's health status. The closed-awareness context of the dying patient likewise reveals further aspects of this process.

7

A Systems Analysis:
Exchange and Equilibrium
in Group Behavior

*E*fforts to understand something as complex as human behavior, both individual and group, have turned to several guiding frameworks derived from other sciences. Early physical theory, especially the Newtonian world view, offered us a machinelike analysis of nature that was all too easily transferred to the realm of the human. Human life was considered to be like a giant machine with mechanical links and connections exercising their direct and clocklike control over the person and society. In time, the Newtonian concepts in physics gave way to a less neat mechanical view of the physical world. New models were introduced to enrich the knowledge of human behavior.

Many of these new models turned away from the physical sciences' perspective and turned to the view emerging within the life sciences. The organic model of nature, derived largely from the study of living biological systems, offered an attractive way of understanding human life. Eventually, this organic metaphor was shaped into a variety of theories, which we will consider under the general heading of systems analysis.

SYSTEMS PERSPECTIVE

When we adopt an organic or biological metaphor, we consider the subject of interest to us (e.g., group process) as though it were a living system. As we know, living systems (also called open, as contrasted with closed systems) are composed of elements that function together and

119

that engage in an exchange relationship with their environments. The human body is such a system: its parts consist of several subsystems that are interrelated (i.e., interact with one another) and that function together to achieve a balance or an equilibrium both internally and in exchanges with the surrounding environment.

The very concept of system suggests parts that hang together, that work together, and are interdependent even though specialized in their function. Thus, if a group is said to function like a system, the parts (i.e., members) behave differently together than when not part of that system we call the group. Likewise, if we consider a group as a system, we are concerned with the ways in which that system achieves a steady state or equilibrium through its exchanges both with its internal environment (i.e., its member-to-member relations) and its external environment (i.e., the groups' relations with other groups, its designated task, the organization within which it functions, and so forth).

The organic metaphor teaches us that in order to understand the activities of the parts, we must first understand their location and function within an equilibrium-maintaining system. For example, we might understand the failure of a kidney to perform its proper function by viewing it within the context of the whole living body of which it is a part. That is, the demand on the kidney was increased leading to its failure because another subsystem of the body failed to function properly. In a similar way, we attempt to understand the behavior of any single group member by viewing it within the context of the living system (the group) of which it was a part. Before we examine the implications of this theoretical perspective, let us first consider several important characteristics that systems contain.

Elements

A system is comprised of elements or parts. A group, for example, contains individuals who are its members. A family contains individuals who are its members. An organization (e.g., a hospital) contains individuals and units that are its elements. Something that may be an element in one system can be considered an entire system from another perspective. Thus, for example, the individual is an element in a group; yet from the perspective of bodily functioning, the individual is the system and the body parts are the elements. Or, from still another perspective, the circulatory system is the "system" and the elements involve heart, lungs, blood, and so forth.

Interdependence

The elements of any system are joined together by a relationship of interdependence. Thus, whatever happens to one element in the system has consequences for other elements of that same system. The actions of one group member, for example, affect the actions of other members of the group. Whenever elements are joined into a system, their behavior is no longer independent. The behavior of any one part is thereby intimately linked to the behavior of all the other parts. Our example in an earlier chapter of the nagging wife and the withdrawing husband is one illustrative case. His behavior is linked to hers and vice versa; they do not function independently once they are together.

Wholistic Functioning

The interdependent elements of a system are organized into a whole and function together as a whole. Furthermore, the whole has properties that no element necessarily has. And these properties or characteristics of the whole affect the behavior of each of the elements of the system. Thus, a group has characteristics that no member of the group possesses. It is commonly noted that the whole is different than the mere sum of its parts. A group can be aggressive and combative, for example, whereas members in isolation from one another are more docile and less aggressive. There is something about their coming together into a group that creates aggression as a property of their group as a whole. By noting that properties of the whole affect the behavior of the elements, we are suggesting that members will take on characteristics in one system that are aspects of that system; in another system, they may behave very differently. The adolescent, for example, may be very friendly and open at home but very aggressive and hostile or withdrawn and unfriendly at school. Parts in different systems are not the same.

Causal Analysis

Given the preceding information, we can see that in order to understand the behavior of any element of a system, we must first understand its location within the system. That is, an element is not the same when it is in a different system. To the teachers, the 14-year-old girl may be aggressive or excessively withdrawn; to her parents, she is warm, open, and friendly. Which one is the true person? Both. She can only be understood in the context of school or home. Likewise, when we try to understand the behavior of any member of a group, we must locate our analysis in the ongoing context of that group. Our causal analysis—that is, how we go about understanding the causes of behavior—requires our consideration of the system or context within which the particular element is functioning.

Equilibrium

One of the major properties of all systems is their tendency to seek some point of balance or equilibrium. This property calls our attention to the ways in which systems restore homeostasis whenever events disturb the ongoing state of balance. Most systems with which we deal are termed *open systems*. An open system is one that receives inputs from its environment and sends outputs back into the environment. Open systems are in an exchange with their environment; they are thereby open to having their equilibrium upset. In the living organism, for example, there is an exchange in which oxygen and other nutrients come in and waste products go out. Balance between this input and outflow is a characteristic of such a system. When that balance is upset, illness results.

In a similar manner, when we consider the group to be an open system that seeks equilibrium, we ask about the mechanism by which that group maintains its equilibrium in the face of changing environmental inputs. A family, for example, may have achieved an excellent equilibrium as long as the wife remains at home and does household chores, the husband is away at work, and the children remain young and in school. That equilibrium can be upset, however, by any number of inputs: e.g., the wife gets a job; the children get older and leave home; the husband loses or changes his job; a severe illness strikes one member of the family; and so on.

Basically, any change threatens the stability of a system and thus is resisted. We can learn a great deal about how a system (e.g., a group or a family) maintains its equilibrium by observing what happens when changes are instituted. In psychiatric practice, for example, it has long been observed that as the identified "sick" member is brought into treatment and threatens to get better, other members of the family may begin to get worse. In other words, the family's equilibrium around the "sick member" is threatened by that person's return to health; this then triggers new mechanisms of adjustment designed to retain the entire system in a state of equilibrium. These mechanisms may take the form of withdrawing the sick member from therapy so as to return him or her to the "sick status," or by another member's developing symptoms of illness, or even by the failure of the equilibrium to be restored and the family's dissolution.

Feedback

The information that is fed into a system (either from the outside or from within) which keeps it steering on its course is referred to as feedback. The information, for example, that a thermostat receives regarding room temperature helps adjust the control mechanism directing the heat to be turned off or turned on. Feedback refers to any information that helps steer, guide, or direct the behavior of a system or its elements. The equilibrium of a system is maintained by virtue of feedback mechanisms. In a group, for example, the leader may help steer the group by providing it feedback regarding its present state with respect to its goals. We discuss this further in Chapter 11.

A WAY OF THINKING

The systems perspective, in this case, is a way of looking at groups. It directs attention to certain aspects of reality; it helps organize our experience and provide us with the tools we need for better understanding. When we speak about the group as a system, we are adopting a perspective that emphasizes (a) how structures and relationships emerge within a group; (b) how they grow and develop over time; (c) how they are maintained at a relatively steady or stable state; and (d) how they are transformed or changed. This perspective directs our attention to the ways in which groups deal with their task and maintenance problems, the ways in which members are recruited and socialized into their particular roles, how decisions are made, how conflict and disagreement are handled, how leadership and authority are exercised, how relationships develop and evolve over time. Let us use a concrete example we briefly mentioned earlier to help illustrate this perspective.

A team of six health professionals, consisting of a physician, a nurse-specialist, a nutritionist, a physical therapist, a psychologist, and a social worker comprise a rehabilitation team to work with Mrs. Watts and her family throughout Mrs. Watts' colostomy surgery and afterward. Their goal is to draw up a plan that will speed her recovery and improve the quality of her life. Their concern is not only with their prime patient, Mrs. Watts, but with the entire Watts family. The nurse-specialist is primarily concerned with helping Mrs. Watts tend to her colostomy so that it will not be a nuisance to her or to her family; the nutritionist's concern is with issues of proper diet; the physical therapist focues on helping Mrs. Watts rebuild her strength; the psychologist works with her and her entire family to help them deal with the various emotional problems that have emerged because of her surgery; the social worker joins the psychologist in this endeavor and in addition is concerned with developing communitywide support services for the Watts family. In working with the entire Watts family, members of the team become aware of a variety of medical and psychological problems other than the colostomy alone. Daughter Amy, for example, has an obesity problem that seems to have been exacerbated by her mother's surgery. Son Tim has been having school problems. Mr. Watts has had difficulty in getting and retaining employment and seems especially resentful of all the extra care, attention, and expenditures that his wife's illness demands.

The Team.   A systems perspective could focus on the rehabilitation team and its activities or on the Watts family and its mode of functioning. If the team were the focus of our concern, then we would focus on such questions as: How is information brought together from the several different sources? How are decisions made about the family's treatment and progress? Who interacts with whom on the team? Who seems to be most and who seems to be least influential in this decision-making process? How effective is this team? Are there arrangements that would improve the team's efforts? How does its organization affect its effectiveness? What developments in the team interactions and communications have occurred as the members have worked together over time? How are points of view that differ from the majority opinion handled? How is conflict and disagreement handled?

The Family.   Our focus, however, need not be restricted to the team of health professionals; we could focus on the Watts family. Many of the same issues and questions would then be of concern to us: e.g., What pattern of interaction and communication characterizes this family? How are family decisions made? How is conflict handled? In what ways are the medical problems expressed within the family? What is the effect on the family of Mrs. Watts' colostomy?

Basically, we would view the family as a system; thereby, we would come to see that the well-being of any member of the family depends on our ability to deal effectively with the family as a whole. We would try to understand, for example, how the daughter's obesity problem and the son's school problem fit into this family's modes of dealing with its medical problems. That is, we would attempt to understand how the multiple problems facing this family weave themselves into a whole, a fabric with its own characteristics. We would adopt this wholistic focus rather than attending to each problem as though it existed in isolation from other problems within the family. The search for the interdependence of parts with the whole, the search for ways in which functions for the whole family are served by the behaviors and symptoms of the members—these are critical aspects of a systems perspective.

How vs. Why

The issues raised in the example direct us to ask questions of *how* more than questions of *why*. Our attention is directed to *how* relationships within groups are formed and *how* these relationships stabilize; *how* decisions are made; *how* patterns of behavior emerge; *how* parts fit together to form the whole family, team, or group (e.g., Lewin, 1951; Spiegel, 1971; Watzlawick et al., 1967).

There is an important distinction between the *how* questions of this perspective and *why* questions as in the psychoanalytic approach. Answers to questions of *why* typically turn toward history or prior circumstances for their answers. For example, if we ask *why* it is that the male psychologist ignores the advice of the female social worker in making recommendations about patient management, we might search for our answer somewhere in his personality, his attitudes toward women, his concerns with status issues, or his understanding of his role as a psychologist. The *how* question tends to turn less toward matters of personal life history for its answer; rather, it deals with present events.

For example, although it may be partly true that the psychologist's reason for ignoring the social worker involves something about his personality and attitudes toward women based on some events in his own past history, our interest is in understanding *how* it is that he presently expresses himself in ways that ignore or reject her opinions and *how* this pattern of relationship influences the entire team's effectiveness. We are less concerned with why he is the way he is and more concerned with how the way he expresses himself affects this team's functioning together.

Kurt Lewin, whose ideas we will shortly examine, had a helpful way of expressing this distinction. He used as illustration the example of a giant boulder poised on the top of an incline; below lies a village in peril if the boulder rolls downward. Lewin suggested that if our concern is with whether or not the boulder will come rolling down, we should care less about why the boulder got to the top of the incline in the first place and be more concerned with its present circumstances. Why it got there is important only insofar as it informs us about the present situation; the present situation, however, will inform us about whether or not the boulder is likely to come rolling down on the village. Notice, a focus on process does *not* ignore the whys; rather, it suggests that complete understanding requires a primary focus on here-and-now processes.

Now that we have the general idea of group process involving a systems analysis, let us add to this theoretic perspective by introducing several exemplars of its use. We will begin with the perspective offered by Kurt Lewin, one of the most significant figures in the study of group dynamics.

LEWINIAN LIFE SPACE THEORY

For us to appreciate fully Lewin's contributions, we must first examine several key concepts that he introduced, particularly, his concept of the life space.

Lewin used the term *life space* to refer to the life world or the environment experienced by the individual or the group. The life space is the world as the individual or group experiences it, their psychological environment. A person's life space might consist of the options that he or she might envision while planning for an evening's activities. In a similar manner, a group can be said to have a life space; this refers to the aspects of the groups' social world that exist for it as it plans its activities and conducts its business.

Lewin noted that the life space represents the world as perceived by the members. He notes that if members fail to include certain items in their life space, then these items cannot exist as determinants of their action. In other words, if a group is developing a care plan but fails to consider certain matters (e.g., including the children of the patient as relevant to her aftercare program), then this option is not included within their life space.

In order to describe the essential features of a life space, Lewin introduced the following set of concepts: *regions, paths, goals and valences, barriers,* and *forces.*

Regions.   A region involves any aspect that is differentiated from the background. Regions include activities, thoughts and ideas, actual places, and such. For example, people attempting to decide between going to a movie or staying home and studying could be said to have two regions in their present life space: the movie and studying. Thoughts or ideas are likewise considered to be regions in a life space. For example, the idea, "If I work hard, I can succeed in life" and the idea, "Success is a matter of luck and who you know" can be considered two regions of a person's life space.

Groups as well as individuals have regions that describe their life space. A group working on a task, for example, may have a definite set of specific activities that must be completed before the task is accomplished. Each activity is a region in that group's life space: e.g., obtain a detailed history from a patient; send the patient in for some blood work; get x-rays taken; do a routine physical examination; meet at the end to pull together the bits and pieces of information; arrive at a diagnosis and treatment plan.

Knowledge of the regions into which persons or groups have differentiated their life space is important if we are to understand not only what they are thinking but also where they see themselves to be at present and what options they see existing for their behavior. As we previously noted, unseen options cannot be taken; they are not represented as regions within the life space. This often can be vital information necessary to our understanding.

Paths.   Paths refer to the linkages or connections between regions. The existence of a path joining two regions indicates that the person or group feels that it is possible to move from one region to the other. The absence of a path suggests that the person or group does not see a way from one region to the next. For example, Susan may be in a decision dilemma, trying to decide among courses for the coming term. She may arrange a listing of several possibilities based on her interests, what is available, and what she is required to take. These comprise the regions of her life space as it applies to the act of decision making. As Sue reviews that listing, however, she notes that taking one course prohibits her taking another; both meet at the same time. These two regions are not connected by a path. Other courses, however, may be connected; taking one is required in order to take another.

Often in helping people or groups evaluate their life space, we encounter a situation in which we think a path exists but they do not. They feel trapped; they fail to see the possible connections between the present position and other alternatives. In a life space analysis, where a path does not exist in the experience of the person or group, then movement is not possible. Only when people see the possibilities for moving from region to region are they likely to make such moves. In the example, we see a path that the others do not see; we see movement possibilities; they feel trapped. Remember, their behavior is a function of their view and not of ours. Our task, therefore, may require helping them to see paths that were not originally part of their life space.

In many instances, the presence or the absence of a path can be described in motivational terms. People may not feel qualified to do certain activities. For them, there is no path between their present region and another. Again, our task may be to help people see paths that they might not otherwise notice.

Goals and Valences. Some regions within the life space are called goals. These are regions toward which or away from which activity is directed. Goal regions toward which people or groups are heading are said to be *positively* valent. Regions are *negatively* valent when there are pressures acting to push away from that direction. It is assumed that the direction in which behavior will actually go is a function of the combined resultant force of these positive and negative pressures. Determining the valence of the regions in a person's or group's life space is important. It informs us about pressures towards or away from those regions.

Lewin posited several situations in which persons are located between opposing positive and negative valences or between all positively or all negatively valent goal regions. One type of situation involves being located between a positively valent region and a negatively valent region. This is relatively easy to resolve; the person or group heads toward the positively valent region and simultaneously away from the negative region. The donkey facing a carrot on one side and the threat of a punishing stick on the other can be expected to head toward the carrot.

A second type of situation, however, is one in which the person or group is located between two negatively valent regions. In this case, there are no carrots, but only sticks. Pressures are for staying put, especially if the negative valence from one side equals that of the other. If, however, the negative push is more intense from one side than the other, the balance will tip the person or group toward the lesser of the two evils.

A third type of situation finds the person or group between two positively valent regions. In this case, pressures are pushing toward movement in both directions. Typically, as the person or group leans one way, this is sufficient to resolve the dilemma and push further in that direction.

It is valuable for the investigator of group process who is attempting to make a life space analysis of the group to inquire about group goals and positively and negatively valent regions. This will be highly informative concerning the likely actions that the group will take.

Barriers. Barriers are obstacles to movement through the life space. These obstacles either make movement difficult or stop it entirely until a way around the barrier can be found. In trying to comprehend the behavior of individuals or of groups it is essential that we understand the kinds and location of barriers that they experience within their life space. Remember, what *we* assume and what *they* assume to be an obstacle may differ substantially; their behavior is a function of their life space as they experience it, not as we think it exists. Thus, when groups or individuals think that barriers exist that prevent them from making the kind of progress they would like, then barriers *do* exist for them. It is up to the analyst of their group process to understand what these barriers are, where they are, and how they may be surmounted if the group is to move forward.

Forces. The concept of *force* is basic to a life space analysis. A force refers to any source of pressure to move. Thus, the intention to work sets up a force on the person to work; but so too does an order from a superior. Forces are of several different types according to their origins. There are *impersonal forces* that originate from within the environment rather than within persons. A windy day that makes driving difficult, for example, could be described in terms of forces on the automobile that derive from the impersonal force of the wind. There are *induced forces* whose origin is other persons or roles (e.g., the boss, the supervisor) that set up pressure on people to behave in a particular manner. Finally, there are *own forces,* those that originate from within the person or the group.

It is important to distinguish between forces according to their source, but especially between *own* and *induced forces*. Basically, induced forces trigger pressure both in the direction requested by the inducer and opposing, resisting forces in the opposite direction. Own forces, by contrast, do not set up opposing *resistance*. Thus, if a supervisor makes a request, this not only sets up a force to comply with that request but is said simultaneously to set up a force toward resisting. If we make the same request of ourselves, however, the resisting component is not created. In a highly cohesive group, members can set up forces on others that have the properties of own rather than of induced forces (see, e.g., Coch & French, 1948). Thus compliance is greater and resistance less. In a less cohesive group, however, commands from one's fellow group members are more like induced than own forces; hence greater resistance is likely.

Resistance does not usually take the direct form of noncompliance. Rather, the presence of two forces in opposing direction (i.e., the induced and the resisting forces) will create a situation in which *tension* is experienced. This tension is usually revealed in many indirect ways, especially in attitude and motivation: persons drag their feet while complying; they fight and complain; they arrive late; they are irritable; they feel resentment; they take little initiative in starting things or in completing things; they require close supervision. Because own forces do not create opposing resistance, these symptoms of tension are not encountered.

Persons who work with groups, especially those interested in helping a group change some of its patterns so that it can become more effective as a working team, will be more successful if they can create own rather than induced forces. We will have more to say about this in Chapter 10 on leadership. For now, however, it is important to recognize that groups (and individuals) tend to resist change that is induced from outside. Helping a group, therefore, without inducing resistance, requires creating a climate in which the group induces its own forces on itself rather than having such forces induced from outside.

Certain intervention styles—for example, democratic and participatory approaches—are likely to minimize the source of resistance stemming from opposition to induced forces. Other styles—for example, more autocratic and unilateral approaches—are more likely to earn compliance that is accomplished by some degree of resistance as well as the symptoms of tension.

To summarize thus far, in order to make a useful analysis of individuals' or a groups' life space (their psychological environment as they experience it) it is necessary to proceed by attempting to determine regions, paths, goals and valences, barriers, and forces. A full understanding of these aspects of the life space will prove helpful in determining why behavior proceeds as it does or why certain actions that one might expect do not occur.

With Lewin's concept of life space in mind, we can look at his application of these concepts to the systems perspective. We can see how his ideas merge with a system's analysis to provide a useful theoretical tool for the understanding of group process.

HERE AND NOW

An important aspect of Lewin's approach, one that clearly stresses the system's perspective, is his contention that it is the contemporaneous life space rather than the past that must concern us: remember his example of the boulder. His focus is on the here and now rather than on past events. In this regard, Lewin's approach and the symbolic interactionist position are similar; both emphasize processes here and now taking place. A life space analysis must attempt to evaluate the configuration of forces that persons feel are relevant to their present circumstances: things now pressing on them; options and choices they experience here and now.

Naturally, those elements of the past that people experience to be present and affecting them right now must be included. Thus, the concentration on the present does not rule out the past; present representations of that past as people experience them make up an important part of their contemporaneous life space. But so too do projections toward the future. Thus, hopes and expectations for the future can be a part of the here-and-now life space.

This "here-and-now" concept is difficult to understand; an example may help clarify it.

> Adele Hamil is a psychiatric nurse who works with two rather different adolescent groups. The first involves some fifteen hyperaggressive boys on an in-patient unit at a hospital; on Sundays, she works with the second group, a relatively normal teen group in her community. She is fortunate in that her circumstances allow her to make comparisons between the processes of interaction in the two groups. She has noted one very significant difference. Whenever one boy in the hyperaggressive unit makes *either* a friendly or an unfriendly gesture to another boy, the other boy's response is the same; he responds aggressively. By contrast, in her teen group, only unfriendly gestures are met with aggressive and unfriendly responses; friendly gestures are met with friendly responses (from Raush, 1965).

What may appear to be a relatively simple, even minor observation actually provides us with a rather potent way of understanding the emphasis on the here-and-now. If both friendly and unfriendly gestures are met with the same unfriendly type of response, this suggests that the hyperaggressive boys cannot differentiate between friendly and unfriendly acts. They respond aggressively regardless of the other person's initial overture. Rather than our asking why they do this, we ask *how* this pattern of interaction affects them and others in their group.

Once we adopt this perspective, we see two things occurring within the hyperaggressive group:

—Once a cycle of interaction is started, regardless of how it begins by either a friendly or an unfriendly overture—it will end up unfriendly.

—This cycle helps reinforce the boys' own hyperaggressiveness; their unfriendly response to a friendly overture provokes an unfriendly reply; this permits them to continue to act aggressively and feel justified in doing so.

The following diagram clarifies this second point:

A   John is friendly to Tom.
   B   Tom's response is to be unfriendly and aggressive to John.
     C   John's response to Tom's aggressiveness is to be aggressive.
      D   Tom's response to John's aggressiveness is to be aggressive.

At point D in the sequence, Tom can justify his own aggressiveness by noting that he is simply doing unto John what John did unto him—returning aggression with aggression. Tom fails to see how his own behavior at point B helps to keep his cycle going.

This example illustrates how a focus on the contemporaneous interaction between persons in the group enables us to understand how an unhealthy, self-perpetuating cycle develops and becomes a stable characteristic of that group. Not surprisingly, in attending to the how question we have come up with an answer to one question of why. The answer to why hyperaggressiveness seems to persist in these boys is suggested by the self-perpetuating quality of their cycle: they feel justified in being aggressive as their response to others' aggressiveness.

This analysis also gives Nurse Hamil some help in intervening in order to facilitate change. Once she has determined the nature of the group's interaction cycle, she is able to break it by refusing to return their aggression with her own aggression. That is, she can curb her own tendency to feel disturbed whenever her friendliness is met with unfriendliness by recognizing that to do so only helps to reinforce the very pattern she must disrupt. To disrupt this unhealthy pattern, she refuses to act on her own feeling but rather replies in a friendly manner to unfriendly responses. Note: she does not seek to intervene in the process by probing back into the history of the causes of the boys' aggressiveness; she works on the here-and-now situation presented to her.

This focus informs us that systems such as this group tend to maintain themselves in a steady state or some kind of equilibrium; in this case, the equilibrium exists around the maintenance of hyperaggressiveness. In the case of a nagging wife and a withdrawing husband, an equilibrium may exist because the pattern of nag-withdraw is maintained. If either partner fails to respond in a way that would maintain that cycle, then it might be broken and the unhealthy equilibrium would become open to change.

Our search for the interconnectedness between obesity, school problems, and the colostomy in the Watts family example is likewise motivated by this same focus. We search for the ways in which the elements of the group fit together and maintain themselves in a relatively stable state. We ask what contribution is served by the daughter's obesity or the son's problem in school to keep the Watts family in a state of relative equilibrium.

In other words, whenever we encounter some relatively stable, ongoing pattern of behavior within a group, a systems analysis demands that we try to understand how that pattern is maintained. Furthermore, it demands that we try to understand how the several parts of the group (i.e., its members and their own individual behaviors) fit into the overall pattern and its maintenance. Finally, it demands that we try to understand how we can intervene to alter the self-maintaining pattern should it be unhealthy or a problem. This then brings us to another feature of Lewin's theory.

THE ORGANIC WHOLE

In outlining the systems perspective, we noted its emphasis on the concepts of interdependence and wholistic functioning. We can now examine these in more detail as Lewin has used them.

The life space does not consist of a set of discrete, independent parts that have little or no connection to one another; rather, it is comprised of a set of regions that are in an interdependent relationship to one another. A change in one part, therefore, has consequences for the rest of the life space. Essentially, one cannot tinker with one element of a life space without thereby causing changes in the other elements. A state of *dynamic equilibrium* is said to exist; pressures arise to restore it whenever something occurs to upset the balance of the total system.

Lewin's analysis can be applied to the life space of an individual as well as to the life space of groups. We can see the individual members of a group as the interdependent regions of a life space; a change in one upsets the delicate balance and leads to pressures to restore the balance. Consider the following examples:

> Nurse Alvarez can always be counted on to lend a light and humorous air to the atmosphere on her unit. In fact, her presence at meetings and informal get-togethers seems to keep the entire group rather congenial and without much conflict and bickering. Tuesday, however, she arrived feeling very depressed. Her entire manner was subdued; she was passive and withdrawn. The group meeting that day was marked by conflicts among several others on the unit; there was a great deal of arguing, petty bickering, and minor quarrels. Even Nurse Alvarez was brought into the fracas as several other nurses "ganged" up on her, becoming highly critical of her techniques for dealing with patients and being especially upset with her apparent passivity and withdrawal.

As we reflect on this event, we suspect that the group was held together in a delicate, conflict-free balance as long as Nurse Alvarez's humorous and mediating behavior siphoned off any undercurrent of tension and hostility that existed. A change in her behavior for that one day, however, resulted in a dramatic change in the entire group. Even she was the recipient of much pressure to become her old self again, as though persons implicitly understood that her old self served a useful function for the group—namely, keeping conflict at a minimum.

> As part of her nurses training, Joy Hartlow observes a family therapy session once a week at a nearby clinic. At this particular session, the mother, the father, and their young son are present along with the therapist, Dr. Watson, and his co-therapist, Ms. Robins, who is a social worker. Joy notices that whenever either therapist addresses the son, either the mother or less often, the father, speaks up, adding her/his own commentary to whatever the boy says. In particular, it seems that every time the boy says

something that indicates that he wants to be relatively independent and do things on his own, his mother makes a comment such as: "Well, he's a bit too young for something like that; we don't want to overprotect him, but he just isn't capable yet of doing very much on his own." The father often concurs with this, but then later is critical of his wife's overprotective way of handling his son. In his view, the boy is capable of many more things than any 9-year-old could possibly do and it is his wife's fault that the boy is "disturbed." Then, the husband and wife begin to argue together over their son and their way of relating to him: the wife objects to the husband's wanting too much from a disturbed child; the husband retorts that the disturbance has resulted because she has not made enough demands on the boy.

In this example, the relationship between the husband and wife is centered around the son and his disturbance. It almost appears as though their son's disturbance is a necessary condition of their marriage and their connection to one another; that is, without a disturbed son, perhaps the family group would not be able to stay together. Therefore, as the son begins to move toward health and well-being, there is apt to be pressure from the father and mother for him to remain ill so that their own relationship can remain intact.

Advice for Practice. In both of these examples, the group functions as an organic whole, a total system with interdependent parts. We fail in our efforts to understand the behavior either of the group as a whole (e.g., the outbreak of frequent petty conflicts in the first group) or of individual members of the group (e.g., the continuation of the young boy's disturbed condition in the family group example), unless we can see these as elements of a total system or organic whole. This aspect of the Lewinian perspective forces us to attend to whole systems in order to understand the functioning of the parts; to focus on the relationships that connect parts together into a whole; to be oriented to *gestalts*—that is, patterns and configurations, rather than separated pieces.

This represents powerful knowledge for the student of group process; it forces a consideration of the larger context within which an individual's behavior occurs in order to understand that behavior. In turn, it likewise necessitates an examination of the larger context within which a group functions in order to better understand its behavior. That is, if individuals can be seen as the interdependent elements that comprise a group, then groups can be seen as interdependent elements that comprise a still larger whole—for example, an organization (hospital, clinic, etc.). Thus, if our understanding of an individual's behavior is enhanced by understanding the group within which that person functions, then our understanding of groups is further enhanced by seeing that group as one part of still larger systems.

Dynamic Equilibrium

The perspective of seeing things in terms of the whole system makes possible an awareness of the ways in which the status quo within a group—the existing patterns of relationship and ways of behaving—is the result of an active process, termed a *dynamic equilibrium*. The family is held together and functions reasonably well as long as the son remains disturbed; or the group is free of conflict as long as one member is present and performing her mediating functions. The student of group process must begin to see the ways in which dynamic equilibrium is maintained; that is, the configuration of forces that press in equal but opposing directions to maintain the status quo.

Thinking in these terms enables us to better understand the behavior of individuals within a group. The behavior takes its form from the characteristics of the group as a whole. Nurse Alvarez was constrained therefore to play her part in mediating conflicts so that the group could continue without change. When she came in feeling depressed, she became the target of others' anger; her depression meant a change in the one element that was necessary to maintain the group's existing level of functioning—i.e., its equilibrium.

Kurt Lewin introduced the concept of *quasi-stationary equilibrium* to explain a group's steady or persistent pattern of behavior (see Lewin, 1947a,b; 1951; Also Coch & French, 1948) as a balance between opposing tendencies of forces. Lewin uses the example of a work group to illustrate the concept. The level of productivity of this group appears relatively stable over a period of several months. In his terms, the level is the resultant of a quasi-stationary equilibrium process. The group's production level is maintained by a balance between factors that lead toward higher productivity (e.g., wages) and factors that lead toward lower productivity (e.g., fatigue).

Lewin next notes what we would do if we were interested in changing that group's level of production. Given a systems analysis, we can do this in two ways: (1) we can add further weight to factors that help increase productivity, or (2) we can reduce the weight of factors that oppose productivity. For example, we could increase wages as a way to add more weight to a factor that leads to greater productivity.

Or we could try to minimize the fatigue that the workers experience, adding more breaks to the work schedule, for example, and thereby reduce the weight of a factor that opposes high productivity. In either case, we try to establish a new level of productivity, a new quasi-stationary equilibrium.

Lewin suggests, however, that one consequence of adding to the weight of factors that increase productivity is to create a higher level of tension within the group. This is not as likely if we try to minimize opposing factors. For example, increasing wages may indeed get people to work harder, but this may in turn create greater fatigue. The conflict between wanting to get the higher wages and trying to avoid excess fatigue can result in tension within individuals and the group as a whole. By contrast, reducing the fatigue that persons experience can lead both to increased productivity and to less overall tension. Reducing fatigue and raising wages might work best of all.

When we began to think of groups as organic wholes, as systems with interdependent parts that function in a state of dynamic equilibrium, then we can see the resistance to change that can exist within groups. This leads to another of Lewin's points, one that we encountered in Chapter 1.

Intervention and Resistance

Lewin's analysis speaks directly to the point of intervention within a group. Resistance is likely when the intervention is directed toward one part of the total without due consideration for the whole. Therefore, one is advised to work with the group as a whole rather than with its separate parts.

We recognize that the parts are linked together into an organic whole, and that the stability of that whole is the result of the relationships among those parts. Therefore we can see that to change any one part in isolation from these connections is to threaten the integrity of the whole. Resistance is much greater than would be the case if one were to work with the whole group. This advice, however, though it stems from the Lewinian life space idea, is more often honored in the breech than in practice.

Dr. Wang is a family doctor, yet she never works with the Atkins family as a unit. She sees the husband, the wife, and the two children, all separately. There are a few occasions, to be sure, in which Mrs. Atkins brings in a child and the doctor works with the two of them; and there are some occasions when both Mr. and Mrs. Atkins are brought into joint discussions with the doctor. But typically, members of this family are seen individually. Dr. Wang is frustrated lately by her inability to get the husband, in particular, to follow her regimen of preventive health care. Most of her advice is agreed to in the office and then not followed later on. Dr. Wang has sought to enlist Mrs. Atkins' aid in this matter. Mrs. Atkins agrees in the office to help her husband follow the doctor's advice, but Dr. Wang has reason to believe that much of what she tells the wife does not find its way into changing the husband's behavior.

Although Dr. Wang is engaged in family practice, she is not practicing in the terms of this Lewinian group dynamic model. She deals with individual parts of the whole family but never works with the family convened as a whole unit. Basically, what happens is that individual behavior is being addressed by the doctor and is not being carried out in action by the patient because the advice fails to deal with the reality of the family as a whole unit.

Mr. Atkins cannot readily engage in preventive health care when the behaviors called for on his part would so transform his role within the family that others would be uncomfortable. They resist his changes and he, sensing their resistance, thus fails to practice proper health care. His change in behavior implies changes in their behavior; and they have never been brought in to consult about these broad, wholistic implications. Clearly, Dr. Wang's efforts at preventive health care for the husband must be directed toward the entire family; ideally it should be convened as a family unit to review, discuss, and evaluate the total set of implications for the family as a whole, of any change in the behavior patterns of one of its members. This point is simple and even self-evident, perhaps, but it is one that is typically ignored.

BALES AND SYSTEMS ANALYSIS

The Bales analysis of task and maintenance functions (Chapter 3) provides another example of a systems perspective and of quasi-stationary equilibrium. Bales suggests that a successful group is one in which both task and maintenance functions are served. He notes that groups that overemphasize one function to the detriment of the other tend to be unstable and less effective. In terms of Lewin's quasi-stationary equilibrium analysis, we could say that generally successful groups have achieved a balance between these two opposing factors. They are relatively equal in the weight they give to task matters and to maintenance matters. Adding to the weight of either factor, therefore, would change the groups level of success.

For example, the delicate equilibrium between task and maintenance functions could be upset if greater demands were made on task performance. These pressures to become more effective in task-related issues will result in an imbalance and hence overall ineffectiveness of the group until equal weight is added to the maintenance issues. The reverse is likewise true. Pressures to focus more on maintenance matters will result in upsetting the delicate balance until equal weight is added to task issues. In other words, a change in one side of the quasi-stationary equilibrium equation that ignores changing the other side results in an imbalance that produces less than optimum effectiveness for the group.

THE WATTS FAMILY AND SYSTEMS ANALYSIS: AN EXAMPLE

We should now be equipped to return to the Watts family and examine its group process using some of the major concepts we have introduced. First, we should think of the Watts family as having achieved a state of equilibrium before the diagnosis of cancer in Mrs. Watts. Although we cannot be certain about the aspects that comprise that equilibrium, we can feel fairly confident in assuming that any intact and functioning group (family, in this case) has achieved an equilibrium among its constituent parts. Second, we note that Mrs. Watts' diagnosis of cancer and her eventual surgery upset the family's equilibrium; it changed her relationship to others in the family as the illness took her away from her usual functions and cast these upon other family members. The husband, for example, may have had to take on maintenance chores (e.g., caring for the children and the house) in addition to his regular task activities. Likewise, the children, Amy and Tim, may have been forced to assume greater independence once their mother's function in this regard was lost because of her illness.

If we think of the family in these terms, then our next task is to examine the possible connections between Amy's obesity, Tim's school difficulties, Mr. Watts' employment problems, and Mrs. Watts' illness. We may discover, for example, that Amy's obesity is her way of dealing with the tension she is experiencing by being suddenly cast into the role of "mother," having to take care of the others in her household. Likewise, we may discover that Tim's school problems, especially if their onset correlates with Mrs. Watts' illness, is a reaction on his part to his mother's problems. Mr. Watts' resentment may be reflected through his employment difficulties. Each of these is a real possibility that cannot be discounted as the rehabilitation team confronts the Watts family and attempts to facilitate Mrs. Watts' recovery. Her own recovery can be helped or hampered by the family's attitudes and reactions to her illness.

Interventions designed to deal with any one of these problems must clearly be based upon an analysis of the family's process. Approaching Amy's obesity, for example, without locating it within the matrix of this family's process would not be appropriately responsive to its bases and thus is not likely to be successful. Likewise, Tim's school problems must be seen within the context of the Watts family, as must Mr. Watts' employment difficulties and the course of Mrs. Watts' own recovery. The task that the rehab team faces, therefore, requires that each member work in concert with the others of the team to design the kind of care plan for the entire family that builds upon a recognition and understanding of its group process.

Using Lewin's ideas of a quasi-stationary equilibrium, we can note furthermore that interventions that simply add pressures to one side of the family's process equation are likely only to increase tension, solving little. Like adding to wages without resolving issues of fatigue, placing pressure on one element of the system without reducing pressure in another will only result in greater overall tension. For example, treating Mrs. Watts without treating her entire family is likely only to worsen an already unhealthy equilibrium. The team's responsibility therefore is to assess the total configuration of factors acting on the family attributable to Mrs. Watts' colostomy; and then to work within that broadened conception of "patient."

Group Process and the Health Professional Team

The same kind of process perspective is applicable to the rehabilitation team in our example as well as to its target group, the Watts family. By now it should be obvious that the management of the patient depends on a fine coordination among the participants of the health team. No one of them possesses the key to Mrs. Watts' health; but together, they can bring their varied abilities and skills to bear to promote her health and the well-being of the family. How they function as a team is critical to how well they accomplish their goal of facilitating her recovery.

If we examine the team with a systems perspective, we will be concerned with how it goes about accomplishing its task. In particular, we will be concerned with the ways in which it gathers the diverse kinds of information that are necessary to develop a treatment plan, the ways in which this information is coordinated and a plan proposed, and the ways in which the plan is put into effect. Each member of the team has access to a different view of the patient and her family. How are these different views brought together? How are they coordinated into a treatment plan? How is that plan actually carried out? How is the plan evaluated? How are modifications introduced?

Each of these questions focuses our attention on the ways in which the team goes about its business, the ways it manages itself in the process of managing the patient. Notice that our questions are concerned with *how* the group—the family, the team—functions in carrying out its business. In the example, the business involves the delicate coordination of diverse specialties; our attention is focused on how this coordination is accomplished. We are interested in getting an answer so that we can work to develop a more effective group process. Fundamentally, it is only through our understanding of the process whereby groups function as they conduct their business that we can hope to intervene when necessary to effect an improved process.

In the particular team of our example, we may discover that the expertise of the nutritionist is being ignored by other team members as a treatment plan is developed. Or we may note that the psychologist's perspective is seen to be irrelevant by the physician and nurse-specialist. The team functions, therefore, by avoiding true team behavior: that is, it is a team in name only but not in actual practice. Once we know how it functions, we can be helpful in improving its operation so that it can become more of a team in practice as well as in name.

Unfortunately, all too often a team approach is introduced only to function as an audience so a physician can practice his or her specialty, while ignoring the input from other team members. If medical problems such as those of Mrs. Watts are really family problems as well, if the course of the patient's recovery is dependent on working with the family system, then surely a real team is required. And we cannot intervene with the aim of achieving that reality until we can determine the process by which the team (or group or family) functions in the first place.

It is one of the critical jobs of the analyst of groups to be attentive to the systems perspective and to a concept such as quasi-stationary equilibrium. Without this perspective and this sensitivity to the factors pushing and pulling at a group and its members, the analyst will not only have missed a key element in understanding the groups dynamics but more importantly, will be unable to be as helpful as he or she might have been for the group.

EXCHANGE THEORY

In order to appreciate a recently popular theoretical approach to understanding individual and group process, we need to join the systems metaphor that we borrowed from the biology of living systems with an economic metaphor that we will borrow from the marketplace. The perspective known as exchange theory (e.g., Homans, 1961; Thibaut & Kelley, 1959) introduces an economic, marketplacelike model to the understanding of human relationships and group behavior. Let us begin by introducing several of the basic concepts employed in exchange theory.

Rewards and Costs.   First, let us assume that social interaction can be divided into a *reward* and a *cost* component. That is, it is meaningful to speak about the rewarding aspects to an interaction and what an interaction may cost. For example, it is rewarding to receive approval from another person, but it is costly to receive rejection. Let us next assume that people are hedonistically motivated; they hope to maximize the rewards and minimize the costs that are involved in their dealings with others.

Outcomes.   Next, we introduce the concept of *outcomes*. Outcomes in this context refer to the difference between the rewards and the costs. An outcome may be more rewarding than costly or more costly than rewarding. For example, if I interact with a person who almost always rejects my ideas and rarely approves of things I have said, then the outcome for me of interacting with this person is likely to be negative—i.e., more costly than rewarding.

At first glance, it might appear that I would be a fool to continue interacting with this person, defying the assumption that I am hedonistically motivated. However, since I continue interacting with him or her, there must either be some concealed rewards or some concealed costs keeping me there. I might find it flattering even to be rejected by so highly esteemed and important a person. Or the costs of stopping my interaction with that person might be too much; I might lose my job, so I remain in what is an unpleasant situation because I do not want the even worse outcomes of unemployment.

Thus far, we have used several exchange theory concepts to suggest that people evaluate the rewards and the costs involved in their interaction with others and attempt to achieve the best outcomes that they can. However, there is more to the theory than these relatively simple points. How do people evaluate the outcomes of a particular interaction? What are the standards people use to judge whether a particular outcome is desirable or undesirable?

EVALUATING OUTCOMES

Two investigators, Thibaut and Kelley (1959; we first encountered several of their ideas in Chapter 2), proposed two kinds of standards that we all employ in order to evaluate the desirability of an outcome. They referred to the first standard as the comparison level (CL); they termed the second the comparison level for alternatives (CL-alt).

Comparison Level

Presumably, we each arrive in a given interaction (e.g., a group) with a level of outcome that we expect to receive. This is our CL; it is based on our past experiences with others and even our fantasies about how others should relate to us. We can picture a CL scale that differs for different people. Thus, some persons may have had a past history of miserable interactions with others and so have come to expect little from social interaction. We would say that their CL is low. Almost any outcomes would fall above their CL; they would experience almost anything as a good outcome. Others, by contrast, may have had a past history of very good luck in interacting with others; they have a relatively high CL. Outcomes must be relatively great to be considered good by these persons.

In the exchange model, outcomes that fall above a person's CL are said to be evaluated as good and desirable by that person; outcomes that fall below a person's CL are said to be negative and undesirable. Of course, in that persons differ in the location of their CL, one and the same social encounter may be evaluated as highly positive and good by one person and highly negative and undesirable by another. A person with a low CL may evaluate even a slight smile of approval as providing a good outcome, whereas someone with a high CL will demand much more than a slight smile before he evaluates the outcome as positive.

Comparison Level for Alternatives

The CL-alt is the standard against which people evaluate their outcomes in one relationship with those that are available to them in alternative relationships. In a sense, therefore, people are like shoppers in the marketplace, judging the outcomes they receive in one shop (e.g., in one group or one interaction) with those that are available in the shop down the street. The important alternative of being alone, in no group or relationship at all, is also considered. In evaluating how good the outcomes are in one group, for example, persons consider not only the outcomes that are available to them in other groups but also the outcomes that are based on being by themselves. People who can provide satisfactions to themselves without others would have a rather high CL-alt. They would have few relationships that provide better outcomes than being alone.

Attraction vs. Dependency

As Thibault and Kelley see it, the relationship between outcomes and the CL and CL-alt provide us with a typology of different kinds of groups. This typology derives from the idea that the CL informs us about how *attracted* a person is to a particular group while the CL-alt informs us about how *dependent* a person is upon a particular group. Thus, outcomes that are above one's CL indicate attraction—the more above they are, the more attractive the group is for the person. Outcomes that are above one's CL-alt indicate dependency; the more above they are, the more dependent the person is on that group, in that few if any equally good alternatives exist. This consideration of attraction and dependency creates the several possibilities that we introduced in Chapter 2. (The reader is referred to that chapter for a specification of these types and some of their implications.)

EQUITY

Another type of comparison of outcomes also occurs; it involves the issue of equity (e.g., Adams, 165; Homans, 1961; Sampson, 1969; 1975; Walster, *et al.*; 1973). The comparison in the case of equity involves examining one's own outcomes relative to the outcomes of other persons in a similar context. In order to understand equity, we need to introduce a new concept, *input* or *investment*.

Recall that outcomes result from the difference between the rewards and costs in social interaction. Inputs or investments involve the things that one puts into a relationship. Hard work and long hours, for example, are investments; so too is seniority or in fact, almost any characteristic that a group, an organization, or a society indicates as something to be considered as an investment worthy of receiving outcomes.

Equity vs. Inequity

Equity is said to exist when one person's ratio of inputs to outcomes is proportional to another person's. For example, if Nurse Smith puts in long hours and works very hard at the job and receives outcomes, in terms of pay and fringe benefits, that are proportional to those of Nurse Jones, who has similar investments of effort and time, then equity is said to exist. As Smith compares his situation relative to Jones' situation, he sees equity; there is a sense of fairness in the way outcomes are allocated.

Inequity exists when the comparison ratio is not proportional; for example, when the outcomes for Smith are either not as great as those Jones receives or if he receives the same outcomes but Smith's investments are greater than those of Jones: e.g., Smith puts in longer hours and gets the same pay as Jones. Inequity implies unfairness in the comparison between members of a group or team or organization. Inequity motivates change. When inequity exists, pressures are created to change the system toward greater equity.

Remedies for Inequity. In the example of Smith and Jones, the inequity could be remedied in several ways. Smith could decrease his work inputs; he could work fewer hours or less hard and thereby reestablish equity with Jones. Or Smith could pressure Jones into working harder and thereby deserve the pay she receives. Of course, Smith could quit or even demand greater pay for his efforts. Basically, the model suggests that persons will act in ways to restore equity when it has been violated; they will attempt to achieve a fairness with respect to what they and others deserve.

An Expanded Application

Issues of equity and inequity are clearly relevant to many working contexts in which the inputs of time and effort or seniority or even sex (equal pay for men and women) and the outcomes of pay and fringe benefits (e.g., having priority in selecting one's own schedule) are highly relevant and often visible. But the equity issue is said to pertain as well to nonwork settings in which investments may include such items as commitment to the group, caring for others, putting in time and effort to the group's tasks. In nonwork interaction, outcomes usually do not include pay but rather the social outcomes of being liked, accepted by one's peers, being respected, and so forth. Again, equity considerations are said to be an important consideration accounting for much of the tension and hostility, or on the positive side, much of the satisfaction, that exists in groups.

It is not unusual to observe a group in which inequity exists and creates considerable difficulty for the group. For example, one member puts in much time, comes to all meetings, takes considerable initiative and responsibility, but receives few of the rewarding outcomes that are available in comparison to others who seem to do less, have less commitment to the group, but yet are more esteemed, more respected, and even more powerful and influential in matters of decision making.

Issues of equity and inequity call our attention to a critical matter for all types of groups, one which the analyst of group process must consider along with the other theoretical issues we have introduced. These issues apply to one's own groups as well as to other groups—for example, families or patient groups. Families are especially prone to inequity issues. Children are forever claiming that they should get privileges that are the same as their siblings or, in many cases, that are the same as their parents: "If you can stay up until midnight, then why can't I?" Likewise, issues often arise within families concerning the equity or inequity that exists if the breadwinner (husband or wife) controls the money and its allocation and the housewife or husband, though investing much in the family, is given little say over family decisions.

Health and Equity

Illness, of course, is an important creator of inequity within groups. A person who is ill is thereby often released from doing his or her fair share. That individual may be permitted to invest less (e.g., in terms of amount of work or effort), while still receiving the same outcomes as others who may even have to increase their own investments to make up for the ill member's reduced load. If inequity creates tension, then we would expect that illness within a group (e.g., a family) should be a source of difficulty. Time would seem to be a relevant issue. Short-term inequity can undoubtedly be better tolerated than longer-term inequity. Thus, a brief illness may create only a small amount of tension; chronic illness, on the other hand, may well prove to be an important source of inequity-based tension.

Because inequity is said to motivate action to reduce itself, we would expect that in some cases the ill member might be motivated to reestablish equity even by working to his own detriment. Thus, the illness could be prolonged as that person continues pulling his fair share when this is not medically warranted. Working with the group and directly confronting the equity issue could prove helpful in such cases. The health professional plays an important role in legitimating illness and the inequity that it usually creates. The professional, therefore, must likewise exercise some responsibility in dealing with the difficulties, both medical and psychological, that result from these inequities.

Equity and Social Comparison

The main dynamic principle of this theory is the idea that persons prefer to be in and to establish equity in their social encounters: that is, inequity motivates tension and change. Practitioners can use this concept to assess tension points within groups and to anticipate issues that are likely to motivate change within the group. Group leaders can use this concept to create a setting in which equity is more likely than inequity: e.g., in arranging work schedules, in dealing with issues of member acceptance or rejection, and so forth.

One of the critical ideas carried by the exchange model is its reminder to us that we are all fundamentally *socially comparative* beings. That is, we do not live in isolation from others; we judge our own worth and the worth of what we do and what we receive by comparing ourselves with others in similar circumstances. This comparative nature gives us our sense of fairness and justice in social relationships. And most of us will react negatively when unfairness results from the social comparisons we make.

Within all organizations or groups that are arranged in some form of hierarchy, in which those at the top get better outcomes than those lower down in the hierarchy, these comparative issues of equity, fairness, and justice are likely to crop up. We can expect that many efforts will be made to provide justifications that indicate why it is equitable for those on top to get better outcomes than those on the bottom or new to the system. Yet we can expect much resentment to develop as well. For example, the new nurse lacks seniority and so is given the worse scheduling. Seniority is taken to be an investment that gives those with it greater privileges over those without it. This justification, however sound it may appear, may nevertheless provoke resentment among those new to the system who in comparing their work and scheduling to others feel that something is basically unfair. We can anticipate that these resentments will gain some form of direct or indirect expression (e.g., the hidden agenda) as members of that unit work together. This is but one example of the ways in which our socially comparative nature links us with others in a process of self-evaluation. And it is one further example of the application of an exchange model to group process.

SUMMARY AND CONCLUSIONS

In this chapter, we have considered a systems analysis using Lewin's life space theory and concepts, Bales' perspective, and the exchange theory of social interaction as illustrations. All systemslike approaches place their emphasis on viewing human interaction and group process in terms of exchange and equilibrium. A system is a functioning whole; its parts function together to establish and sustain a balance or equilibrium in the face of ever-changing inputs, both internal (from within the system) and external (from shifting relationships with the external environment). The systems perspective interprets the functioning of parts only by reference to their place within the context of the larger whole or system; it notes the exchanges that occur between the parts as well as between the whole system and its surrounding environment. Finally, it views the entire system as an attempt to establish and maintain a state of equilibrium between opposing forces and points of tension.

8

Theories of Group Development:
Temporal Relationships
in Group Behavior

*A*s we now know, groups are not static things to be characterized as we might describe a still photograph; the interactions among people wax and wane, take this turn and then another. Our theoretical concepts freeze the moment on a slide so that we may examine it better. Yet the life of a group is one of process, of growth, of movement, of change. The question, of course, is whether some patterning and order exists for these movements and changes through time. We are able to speak about the stages of an individual's growth and development. Are there particular *stages* or developmental periods through which groups also pass as they conduct their business? In this chapter we will introduce several efforts to understand the developmental life process of groups. We will not restrict ourselves to any one theoretical perspective on development, but rather will examine what those people of various theoretical persuasions have had to say.

BALES

Bales was especially interested in understanding the small work group that was given a specific problem to solve and a somewhat limited time in which to accomplish a solution. His observations of the patterning of interaction led him to conclude that groups pass through three critical developmental stages, each of which focuses on a specific question (Bales, 1955).

ORIENTATION ASKS: "What is the problem"?
EVALUATION ASKS: "How do we feel about it"?
CONTROL ASKS: "What should we do about it"?

149

To speak of these three as developmental stages is to suggest that whenever a group comes together to deal with a problem, it must confront each of these issues in turn, and answer each of these questions in turn, in order to move toward a solution.

Let us be clear about this matter. One group member may reverse the ordering, trying first to deal with the issue of control even before the problem has been clarified. Another may focus on evaluative issues before considering the dimensions of the task at hand. In other words, this model of development calls our attention to a stagewise developmental sequence that *in general* will characterize successful problem solving in groups. Individuals may wish to skip stages, but in due time the group will have to return to deal with the prior issues.

In this respect, this developmental model for groups has its parallel in developmental models of individual growth. Adolescents, for example, may wish to rush headlong into the issues of the adult world and bypass those of their own age; yet in time, those earlier issues will have to be dealt with. For example, adolescents may wish to move into an intimate, long-term relationship with another person before they have satisfactorily confronted the prior issues of identity. A safe bet is that the fling at intimacy will not succeed until they make some headway in negotiating the prior issues of identity.

Much the same idea can be applied to Bales' three stages of group development. To attend to stage two issues of evaluation or stage three matters of control before even orienting the group to the nature and dimensions of the problem will only delay dealing with the prior matter. As we will see in the chapter on leadership, a group leader, aware of these stages of development and skillful in diagnosing a group's present location along this sequence, can prove helpful in redirecting a group and thereby facilitating its development. That is, the leader can help the group pass through its normal developmental sequence by returning members to earlier issues if they deal with later issues out of their proper sequence. The member who wishes to focus on control when the problem has not yet even been clarified can be helpfully redirected to begin with first things first.

TUCKMAN

In 1965, Bruce Tuckman attempted to synthesize the major literature on group development. He suggested that four developmental stages characterized most of the theories he reviewed. Basically, as with Bales' scheme and as with the others we will consider, each stage represents *an issue* that the group must consider and resolve in order to move successfully forward to the next stage. Tuckman outlines the following four stages:

FORMING: This is similar to Bales' idea of orientation. All groups must initially deal with the issues of coming together, of forming into a group. These involve dealing with who the people are, what their resources and talents are, what the task is, how they might work on it.

STORMING: Somewhat similar to Bales' evaluation stage, storming involves the formation of subgroups that tend to produce conflict, disagreement, and polarization over the task and how it should be done and over the desirable relationships among the members. Conflicts and disagreements over group leadership and the exercise of authority also arise and characterize this phase of group interaction.

NORMING: Once the conflicts have been resolved, the group begins to develop norms and rules to govern its activities. In this stage, we see the beginning sense of the group as a cohesive unit facing a common set of problems that require joint effort to solve.

PERFORMING: This is similar to Bales' control phase. It involves the group's actual work on the task at hand.

It is important for the student of group process to reflect for a moment on the stages that Tuckman has summarized. In particular, the presence of a stage of conflict is important to consider. In this view, conflict and disagreement over task and personal issues is seen to be a normal developmental stage that all groups must pass through before they can get down to the business of doing the actual job for which they have convened. Conflict, therefore, is not inevitably destructive nor a symptom of a faulty group; in fact, it is something to deal with and to build upon.

A group that jumped from forming to norming, for example, refusing to deal with the underlying disagreements that exist whenever persons are convened to work together, might initially appear happy, harmonious, and in agreement. Yet one would suspect that its underlying disagreements and conflicts, never having been confronted directly in the storming phase, would emerge in many subtle and not-too-subtle ways perhaps to sabotage the group's effectiveness in performing.

The group leader would do well to consider these normal stages of development. In particular, it is useful to hypothesize that the absence of a storming period does not mean, "I've got a good group." It may mean that something is inhibiting members' expression of their disagreements; this is not a good sign for the group's long-term work together. Likewise, a group leader would do well not to shudder and abandon all hope should the normal period of storming occur. Needless to say, we are not encouraging the wholesale abandonment of reason to full-fledged storming. We are encouraging persons to consider very carefully the implications of a developmental model of group process in which storming is considered part of the normal growth process and not an aberrant tendency.

SCHUTZ

William Schutz (1960) developed a theory of interpersonal needs, a test to measure those needs, and a conception of group development that built upon both. The theory is similar in many respects to the psychoanalytic model which parented it. Schutz suggests that all persons have what he terms interpersonal needs; these are needs that can be satisfied only by and with others. They are said to be three in number: *inclusion, control,* and *affection.* Each involves a particular issue or set of related issues. Inclusion involves the issue of belonging, of being in or of being out, of bringing others in or excluding and rejecting others. Control involves issues of authority, of dominance and of submission. Affection involves issues of intimacy, of closeness, of caring, of disliking, of distancing.

Schutz's developmental theory argued that these three interpersonal needs, in the I-C-A order (inclusion-control-affection), describe the developmental stages that groups pass through in coming together and working together. He further suggested a point that the other theories we have considered have ignored—namely, a developmental sequence for the *termination* of a group. Here, he indicated that the termination order reverses the original sequence and takes the form of A-C-I. Let us briefly examine each of these in turn.

Forming

The I-C-A developmental pattern suggests two important matters: first, the critical issues that groups must confront; second, the ordering with which these issues are faced. In this respect, Schutz's concept of group development is similar to all concepts of development: a set of critical issues or critical stages is introduced and an ordering to these is provided.

Inclusion. The first issue confronting a group involves *inclusion*. Somewhat similar to both orientation and forming, inclusion focuses on the issues of membership and commitment. It is said that groups must consider who the members really are, who is committed to the group, who rightfully belongs, and who is present but not a true member.

It might sound strange to speak about inclusion as an issue for most work groups; after all, the membership is assigned by the work setting and thus presumably everyone who is said to be a member of the group or the team is a member. Thus, supposedly the inclusion issue is handled formally and thereby, in this view, surely cannot be an issue for the group. On the contrary, inclusion remains an issue to be considered by the group even when a formal assignment of members has been made. Inclusion also deals with the more subtle kinds of in-out relationships, especially those involving different levels of commitment to and involvement with the group as a group. Formal and nonvoluntary work groups are especially prone to inclusion issues; after all, people were simply thrown together and implicitly told to be a group. Yet this is not sufficient to make them a group until they can focus on the inclusion issues, especially the more subtle meanings of membership and commitment.

Control and Affection. The issue of control, the next in the developmental sequence according to Schutz, focuses on the critical theme of authority, dependence, and autonomy. These are all issues with which we are familiar from the psychoanalytic perspective (Chapter 5). Recall that the dual issues of authority and intimacy are critical to all groups. What Schutz suggests, following the general outlines of the psychoanalytic model, is an ordering, a developmental sequence to these two issues: issues of control and relationships with authority are said to precede issues of affection and intimacy. It is as though one cannot begin to relate on a basis of equality within the group, to explore more fully with one another the various kinds of attractions and repulsions that exist, until one has first dealt with matters of control. These tend to differentiate and often stratify members into the more and less powerful or influential; and until this is dealt with, other aspects of member relationships, involving attraction and intimacy, cannot be confronted as directly.

Terminating

In terminating, Schutz suggests that groups pass through these same stages but in a reverse order. Thus, the first issues that come before the group as they head toward their termination involve the bonds of attraction that were involved. Next, issues of control are considered; and finally, inclusion, as the group or the relationship ends.

Keep in mind that these issues will not always be as openly expressed as our description suggests. As we observe a group in action, we will not inevitably witness persons speaking directly about "inclusion" or "control" or "affection." What we must learn to do, therefore, is to inquire and to probe beyond the surface manifestations and content that is directly discussed; we must look for symptoms of these underlying themes and issues and ask ourselves if an understanding of such issues helps us better comprehend what is taking place in the group.

An Example.   When a group convenes for the first time and we observe its interaction, the word "inclusion" will probably never be spoken; people may not discuss commitment to the group, who is in and who is out, what it means to be a member of this group, and so forth. People may only talk about job-related issues, concerning a particular patient, for example. There will be different rates of participation in the discussion; there may even be some disagreements; certain persons may seems more involved and interested in the discussion, while others may seem more withdrawn into their personal issues, or bored with what is happening, or talking on seemingly irrelevant matters.

If we study this group with the Schutz scheme in mind, inclusion is likely to be discovered as an underlying issue that will help explain many aspects of what we observe; members will express in various ways (not always explicitly) their different needs for being included, their fears about being a member and committed to the group and to others, their desires to bring in or include others, and so forth.

We would suspect that inclusion issues are relevant and are being dealt with in often subtle and indirect ways. We would also expect that individual differences in commitment to the group, as evidenced for example in different amounts of participation and concern for the group's welfare, are important matters for the group to deal with openly and directly before such inclusion issues become hindrances to the group's working effectiveness. A leader of this group would use his or her theoretical sensitivities to this possibility to help facilitate the group's dealing with whatever issues and conflicts arise over, in this instance, inclusion and commitment. Members' attention may even have to be focused on their differences in apparent contribution and involvement in the group. Do these reflect differences in commitment to the group? Are these differences proving troublesome to the group's operation?

Basically, the developmental theory can be used as a tool to help guide our understanding and our intervention; it provides us with a useful interpretative framework for putting together what would otherwise be discrete bits and pieces of observed information. But, most importantly, the developmental models generate hypotheses about what may be taking place; thereby they help us work more effectively with the group.

Of course, these are just hypotheses, tentative proposals and interpretations, not facts carved in granite. Thus we must remain open to the possibility that what the theory suggests is happening or should be happening, may not be. But without a theoretical tool, we could not even formulate clear hypotheses about what was taking place and thus not even be able to prove ourselves to be wrong about what we see. A good theory, therefore, lets us know when we are wrong as well as helping to guide us in more correct directions.

SLATER AND BION

For the final developmental approach, we will briefly examine a rather complex model, evolving from a psychoanalytic base and focusing on group development as a function of different ways of coping with underlying basic anxiety. This model can be attributed both to Bion's pioneering work, aspects of which we considered earlier (Chapter 5), and to the observations and interpretations that Slater more recently proposed (1966); it also shares much with the works of Bennis and Shepard (1956). As with other conceptions of group development, Bion's and Slater's work focuses on the critical issues that a group faces and the time sequencing in which these issues are likely to be confronted.

Engulfment vs. Estrangement

In many respects the Slater-Bion model is unlike the previous approaches we have considered; it attempts to understand the surface features that we observe in terms of a deep-lying tension that presumably exists within all persons. This tension derives from the opposition between two tendencies. The first is to join, to merge, to commit, to become one with, to lose one's independent identity. This can be termed *deindividuation* or *engulfment*, a loss of one's individuated identity. The second tendency is to separate, to become unique, to be apart from, to be an individual. This is referred to as *individuation* or *estrangement*, the creation of a clearly separate individual identity.

As described, these two tendencies are in opposition; one cannot simultaneously have it both ways. It is not possible to simultaneously individuate and deindividuate, merge with and separate from. A tension exists, therefore, as people swing between these two extremes. We try to individuate ourselves from others and as we succeed we then feel too much apart, too unique, too alone; thus we try to become like others, to merge with them, to blend into the group, to lose our individuality. But then we fear this loss of our unique identity, and so we begin to move again toward an individuated separateness. Group life makes the tension apparent; we swing between joining and submitting ourselves to the group, and separating, becoming apart from the group. Anxiety is experienced whenever either extreme is approached.

Coping with Anxiety

What the Slater-Bion theory next suggests is that the developmental story of a group can be understood in terms of the different ways in which the anxiety created from these two opposing tendencies is collectively handled. This is an important point. We begin with two fundamental and opposed human tendencies: estrangement and engulfment. We assume that as persons move too far in one direction or the other, these tendencies create tension and anxiety within them. We next assume that there are collective, usually unconscious, strategies and techniques that evolve within groups to cope with this tension and anxiety. And finally, these different strategies give us a developmental sequence for understanding group process. In its early history, groups deal with their basic anxieties with primitive techniques; in time, they develop more "advanced," even productive approaches to handling these basic tensions. This developmental sequence involves the following: fight-flight, dependency, and pairing. We will consider each of these strategies in turn.

Fight-Flight. Early in its history a group has only fairly primitive ways of coping with the anxiety and tension that derives from the estrangement-engulfment tendencies. These relatively primitive methods, which characterize human infants and most animal species, involve either fighting or fleeing. When fight or flight becomes a common mode of functioning within a group, we suspect that the underlying issue involves either the anxiety of estrangement or of engulfment. When a group spends much of its time in conflict and disagreement, and it is either early in its life together as a group or some regression to an earlier mode has occurred, this is reason to suspect that underneath this climate of fighting is a worry that members have either about giving themselves up to the group or of being too separated from the group.

Basically, in this developmental model, fighting behavior within the group is understood as a way members have of dealing with their fears of becoming involved and committed group members or of never becoming involved and having no group exist. To many persons, the former implies losing their individuality; in an effort to keep their uniqueness, they fight and they disagree, as though to proclaim, "See, I am different than you, I think differently, I speak differently, I disagree." Fighting becomes a vehicle for dealing with the fear of engulfment; it involves vociforously proclaiming one's differences from others.

But too much fighting frightens as it separates persons. Thus, an alternative is to flee from the tension and the anxiety by psychologically or at times physically leaving the field of battle. This approach is often reflected when members cannot stick to a given topic and discuss it thoroughly; rather, topics and ideas rush about as though persons do not wish to probe or explore anything too deeply. And when a problem issue arises, members may change the topic or withdraw into some private daydreaming, or begin reading, or engage in what are termed "out-of-the field" activities: i.e., behaviors such as reading that take the person out of the group even while they are physically present.

Dependency. Dependency involves some admission of weakness and a submission of oneself to outside guidance. In groups, dependency is a common strategy for coping with tension and anxiety; it usually takes the form of yielding to a leader or dominant individual. Slater considers this to be a developmentally more advanced approach to handling anxiety. Rather than simply fighting or fleeing, the group turns to someone to help and to guide them. The leader represents someone who will help protect persons from either too much estrangement or too much engulfment.

It is important to note that dependency may focus on a specific person who is the formal group leader, on a specific person who emerges as dominant and protective, or, and this is critical, on anyone or anything that provides structure and organization.

Thus, a group may continually refer to its past meetings and its own history together, using its past as a source of dependency; or a group may refer to some outside authorities or figures on whom it can depend and to whom it can turn for guidance. Likewise, a set of rules or guidelines may become the target for dependency. In all cases, the underlying theme is "we are weak and frightened and need someone or something to nourish us and to provide us a safe structure within which to function."

Even counterdependency—that is, the active rejection of a leader or authority—can be interpreted as an effort to provide structure and protection. The rebel requires the authority figure as much as the conformist. Conformists need to know what the authority thinks so that they may know what they should think; but so too do the rebels. If the authority says yes, the rebel's negative position is thereby clearly defined. In both dependency and counterdependency, the common theme is to invest oneself in someone else who will provide the answers and the structure necessary to stave off the fears and anxieties that would otherwise be present.

Pairing.   In pairing, the third developmental phase in this model, the group has revolted and abandoned its utter dependency on the leader; it is again subject to the potentially devastating fears of estrangement-engulfment. In its search for a suitable way of dealing with these anxieties, it turns to what Bion and Slater refer to as the "unborn leader."

The term "pairing" derives from the observation that groups often break down into smaller subgroups, even pairs of members, who seem to engage in a more intimate and close relationship to one another than to the group as a whole. This intimacy becomes a vehicle for handling the underlying fears and tensions; persons hope that out of their close and warm relationships together they will create a leading figure who will protect them from their dual fears of engulfment or estrangement. Thus pairing, the development of closer bonds between members, becomes a way of dealing with the same underlying issue that has been assumed to motivate the other developmental stages.

In this perspective, it is fitting that pairing should follow dependency. The outcome of dependency is revolt and rebellion against the

leader and authority. This produces considerable fighting and separation within the group, opening it up to the fear of becoming too separate and too estranged, even of dissolving as a group. Thus, to join
hands in pairing is an appropriate reunification, a protection against
too much separation and too much estrangement.

Summary. What Slater and Bion have provided us is a rather
complex, psychoanalytically based analysis of group development in
terms of defensive strategies for dealing with the fundamental anxiety
that derives from the fear of estrangement on the one hand and the
fear of engulfment on the other. Thus, fight, flight, dependency, and
pairing are envisioned as collective ways that groups have for dealing
with the tensions that develop. A never-ending cycle of defensive strategies is posited; the tensions coming from these deep layers of human
existence are never fully resolved. Our understanding of them and
their functioning, however, can help minimize their potentially destructive impact.

In this view, fear of engulfment and fear of estrangement will not
fade from group interaction. The unconscious defensive strategies of
fight, flight, dependency, and pairing will always be present in some
degree or another. A good group, however, is able to work with the
knowledge of these tendencies and defenses to become more effective
rather than crippled and self-destructive. Leadership is especially critical. We turn our attention to this in the following chapters.

SUMMARY AND CONCLUSIONS

An analysis of theories of group development provides us with additional tools by which to understand and to intervene effectively in
group process. All developmental theories offer us two related points:
(1) each outlines the critical issues that are said to confront all groups;
(2) each outlines the particular sequence or order in which these issues
are said to occur. Not surprisingly, whatever the particular persuasion
of the theory, most approaches suggest that issues centering around
authority and leadership on the one hand and around member-to-
member relationships on the other will prove central to all groups.
And most theories locate these developmentally in the sequence: authority issues precede peer relations.

The theories vary primarily in what else they see going on within
groups. From Bales and Tuckman, we see the emphasis placed on task

issues: e.g., defining and clarifying the purposes, tasks, and goals before dealing with matters of actual work and control. From those with a more psychoanalytic bent (e.g., Schutz, Bion, and Slater) we see the emphasis placed on interpersonal issues: e.g., dealing with members' underlying anxieties about the group and their relationship to it.

It is important to keep in mind that all developmental concepts have an ordering that repeats itself throughout the life of the group. That is, a particular developmental stage or issue is never fully completed for all time; rather, as circumstances change, the same developmental issue may crop up again and again. For example, using Bales' analysis, problems of orientation will present themselves again within the life of the group whenever the task changes or whenever a new problem emerges to be dealt with. Or, to use Schutz's model, inclusion will be an issue whenever members change (some old members leave and new members enter the group) or even when the task itself changes and a new kind of group formation may be necessary.

In light of the preceding, it is best to think of a developmental *spiral* rather than a developmental line. A line suggests a beginning and a definite end. A spiral suggests a continuing turn around and around similar issues; it also suggests progress and growth at the same time. Thus, the issues of orientation or of inclusion, for example, will appear again within the life history of a group; but their second appearance will not be the same as their first; nor will the third be exactly the same as the second, and so forth. In other words, the model of a spiral suggests similar issues that are dealt with in somewhat different ways each time they reappear within a group.

This way of thinking is not unusual. Adults often confront issues that are similar to those they faced when they were children; yet, though the problems may be the same, adults do not simply duplicate their childhood ways of dealing with issues. For example, as children, we all faced our first day in school: a new situation and new people to orient ourselves to. As adults we often also face new situations with new people. And again, issues of orientation are relevant. However, we tend to orient differently as adults than we did as children. Much the same can be said of the developmental stages within groups; thus a spiral rather than a line is the best way of representing these stages.

The lessons of group development are important for the group leader. Often, the only sense that can be made out of a given kind of interaction is found through an understanding of the developmental issue that is involved. Furthermore, leader interventions require an understanding of normal group development. Timing of interventions is something that is especially linked to an understanding of development. To push a group too fast toward a later stage when it is still caught up in early-stage issues, for example, does the same to the group that it can do to the individual: i.e., it confuses, leads to resistance, creates frustration, and produces needless tension and conflict.

Assessment and Intervention:
Concepts and Skills
of Group Leadership

Most people using this book are, or will be at some time, group leaders and organizers. The four chapters of this unit are written from the perspective of the leader and with the leader's tasks in mind. The information and ideas, however, are also applicable to group members. When members consider the tasks, issues, skills, and functions of leadership, individuals can become better members. Furthermore, observers who wish to understand group leadership and performance will benefit from the ideas and concepts examined in this unit.

Our aim in this final unit is to build upon the base of previous conceptual and theoretic knowledge in order to facilitate learning the skills of effective assessment and intervention. When health professionals face their first group, it is likely that some anxiety, confusion, doubt, and puzzlement will be present. What do I look for? How do I assess what is taking place? How do I intervene effectively to guide, direct, and lead? What do I do if problems arise? Although the answers to these questions are not simple and do not follow a "cookbook" format, there are some strategies of assessment and leader intervention that can be learned and applied.

In Chapter 9, we consider some approaches for assessing group process. Our eyes and ears still remain our best tools for observing human interaction and small group process. We need to understand where to look and how to listen; we have to know the important ways that people interact and how we can learn to be accurate in our assessment. Both verbal and nonverbal behaviors are addressed in this chapter.

Chapter 10 introduces the topic of group leadership. It discusses the alternative possibilities and styles available to the prospective group leader. We believe that only when group leaders are familiar with their leadership options, can they act intelligently in their group. In this chapter, we examine different styles of leadership and its effects on the members, leaders, and on the group's effectiveness.

Chapter 11 discusses the techniques that groups leaders can learn to become more effective in their leadership role. Although we have a long list of useful intervention techniques, our intent is not to have people mechanically learn a set of rules and unreflectively plug them into the group. These intervention techniques are discussed within a framework that deals with "processing" and with "member resistances." Basically, this framework draws the leader's attention to the living, changing substance that is the group. The group requires continual monitoring and the sensitive use of what would otherwise be merely mechanical routines. When leaders "process" their groups' ongoing interaction and pay attention to "members' resistances" then these intervention techniques are no longer lines to be read without feeling or awareness, but are approaches to reflective intervention.

Chapter 12 confronts some of the major group problems that health professionals are likely to encounter. Seven typical problems are considered: dealing with members who dominate and monopolize, dealing with silence, dealing with emotional displays, dealing with conflict, dealing with normatively deviant behavior, starting a new group, and terminating a group. The purpose of Chapter 12 is to present these problems within the context of a five-stage intervention model: issue, observations, diagnosis, intervention, and evaluation. The model directs the leader's attention to a set of questions to be asked and answers to be sought as an approach to effective intervention.

9

Observational Approaches to Assessing Group Process

*I*t is axiomatic to state that before health professionals can work effectively with groups, they must be able to assess and to evaluate the crtitical characteristics of group structure and process previously considered. In this chapter, we will introduce some of the general observational approaches involved in this assessment.

All of us function within groups; many thereby believe themselves to be intuitively expert about how groups function. However, it takes training and experience to properly and confidently assess this world of our everyday group interactions. In fact, it is the very common-sense quality of our social world that erroneously leads many to believe themselves to possess expertise without need for further direction or training.

We practice what one psychologist has referred to as "bubbapsychology" (McGuire, 1969), using the timeworn homilies of our grandmothers to deal with others. Unfortunately, those intuitive, grandmotherly bits of advice may guide us in opposite directions. For example, one piece of advice to a parent or a group leader suggests that if you "spare the rod you will spoil the child." However, we also learn that "you can catch more flies with honey than with vinegar." So, should the leader be stern and harsh or sweet and kindly? Grandma never tells us everything.

The same bubbapsychology can lead us astray as well when it comes to assessing group process. What are we to conclude when we look at a group of people some of whom are talking, sometimes all at once; others of whom are silent, sometimes all at once? It is difficult enough to know what to look for or at when we attend to one person. But a group . . . ? What we need to develop is a knowledge of some of the major concepts and approaches to group observation that we can systematically employ to sharpen our understanding and to make our intuitive, personal experiences more useful for our daily practice.

OBSERVATION VS. INTERPRETATION

The best tools health professionals possess for assessing groups are their own eyes and ears. It will be helpful to examine some of the general approaches available for observing group and individual behavior. But first, note that we are referring to *systematic* observation. This is to emphasize the point that it is best to observe according to some system rather than in a haphazard or casual manner. We separate what we see or hear from the inferences and interpretations we make based on these observations. For example, we see a smile and infer happiness. We attempt to record and note actual behaviors. We employ known systems for our observations or develop our own systematic framework for the particular purposes at hand.

The point is critical. It is important for observers to be able to separate what they actually see or hear from what they interpret that observation to mean. We do not see anger as such; we do see various behaviors that can lead us to infer anger. For example, Dr. Jones raises his voice above its previous conversational level. He clenches his hands and appears to make a fist. He moves about in his chair, pushing it back from the table; his gestures become larger and more expansive. His face reddens somewhat and his lips become tight. As we listen to *what* he says, we note that the content involves his defense of an intern's right to observe a special procedure even before there has been a detailed study of it. A legitimate inference is that Dr. Jones is angry.

One of the best ways for students to develop their own ability to separate observations from interpretations and to insure that they will be systematic rather than casual about this process is to use a recording form such as the following:

Behaviors Seen or Heard	*Interpretations and Inferences*
1. M. smiles.	1. M. is happy.
2. Dr. Jones raises his voice; clenches his fist; makes large gestures; speaks in defense of an intern.	2. Dr. Jones is angry.

One of the clear advantages to working with such a format is that it gives observers a record of the actual behaviors on which they based their inferences. No comparable record would exist if observers simply recorded interpretations but failed to systematically present the behavioral data on which those were based. Without this record, it is not possible for someone else to evaluate the observations; nor is it possible to test and validate an analysis.

Often it is necessary to gather observations over time in order to test and confirm or disprove an interpretation of behavior. When these observations have been systematically obtained the interpretations can be tested; preliminary analyses can be reevaluated in the light of later observations. This cannot be done, however, if there is no systematic listing of actual observations separated from early or preliminary interpretations.

Let us take an example to sharpen this point. We are observing a health professional team discussing a case and disagreeing about the treatment plan. One member of the team, a recently graduated RN, speaks very softly with the use of many pauses and "uh" sounds that typically indicate anxiety (Kasl & Mahl, 1965). She sits back in her chair, almost withdrawing from others in the group. Most of what she says indicates agreement with whatever anyone else says. We record these observations and our preliminary interpretation: "Nurse Smith appears to be anxious; she is eager to please and to gain acceptance." We may even feel very confident about our interpretation, knowing that she is a recent graduate and that this is her first real work on a team of this sort.

We continue to observe the group's interaction. Later in the same session, we observe the same nurse. Now her manner is more vocal. She speaks much more loudly and in rapid bursts; the pace of her speech has picked up considerably. She has lost the hesitations that characterized her initial conversations. She leans forward in her chair; her gestures have become larger and more expansive. What she says has also changed. She now openly argues and disagrees with the others. Our interpretation as we now observe her is that Nurse Smith seems angry and upset with the group.

We now have a listing of two sets of observations and two somewhat disparate interpretations. We still do not have enough material on which to base a conclusion; however, we do have a relatively firm base of behavioral observations on which to test out one of the competing analyses of Nurse Smith's behavior. Several possibilities exist. We could test each interpretation by directly intervening and asking her a question: e.g., "I've noticed that your manner has changed from early in this session when you spoke hesitantly and sat back in your chair to the present, when you are speaking more forcefully and even argumentatively. I was wondering what this change might mean." Or we might decide to gather more behavioral observations in order to confirm or disprove one of these interpretations or even to develop a different analysis of her behavior and its meaning.

Whichever approach we adopt, it is important to note that they are both built upon our having first systematically distinguished between observations and interpretations. This has permitted us to recall to Nurse Smith her actual behaviors as well as our interpretations and thereby to provide her some behavioral basis for our intervention. This has also provided us with a listing of behaviors and preliminary interpretations that we now have available for later confirmation or refutation.

Types of Observational Data

Basically, there are two types of material available for systematic observation: nonverbal and verbal. Nonverbal observation deals with the mannerisms, gestures, spatial arrangements, touching, intonation, and other such qualities of a person's or a group's behavior. Verbal observation involves both the actual *content* of what is said and the *forms* by which the communication occurs. Content involves what is said, what the people are actually talking about. Form has to do with word choices, use of language (e.g., colloquial or more formal and/or technical), address forms that are used, and so forth. For purposes of assessing group process, we are interested in all of these sources of information. We will begin our analysis with a consideration of the observation of nonverbal behavior.

OBSERVING NONVERBAL BEHAVIORS

Even in our silences we communicate. We who spend so much of our lives talking and trying to choose our words carefully, too often forget the critical role that nonverbal behavior plays in communicating with others. Verbal behavior tends to be more readily under a person's control than the less easily managed nonverbal forms of communication. Sensitive observation of the non-verbal, therefore, can be a potent assessment tool for understanding individual and group process.

Perhaps no profession is more engaged in the observation of nonverbal behavior than the medical and health professions. Persons are taught to observe the slightest change in skin color, for example, as an indicator of possible respiratory disorder. Health professionals note restlessness, body posture, hand gestures, and voice quality (e.g., intonation) to help clarify their medical diagnosis. How often, however, do health professionals observe these nonverbal behaviors in order to determine psychological and interpersonal functioning? Much can be learned about individuals' psychological state (e.g., Are they anxious, depressed, angry?) and about a group's interpersonal state (e.g., Is group morale high or low? Is the group cohesive? Is there conflict within the group?) through observations of nonverbal behavior. For convenience, it is possible to map out several types of nonverbal behavior that are open to our systematic observation and analysis. These include tactile, proxemic, kinesic, and paralinguistic.

Tactile

Tactile communication involves the sense of touch. Individuals as well as cultures vary extensively in their use of touching in communicating. In the United States, for example, males usually do not embrace as a form of greeting; in many Eastern European and Latin American cultures, on the other hand, the embrace between males is not unusual (Jourard, 1968). Some families are high in their tactile communication—children are frequently held, caressed, and touched by parents; family members walk together arm in arm, embrace during times of sorrow and times of great joy. Other families, by contrast, rarely physically touch—children learn to avoid touching other than the few formal gestures, such as handshakes, that most of us have learned. Anyone involved with patient care realizes that touching can be a potent form of reassurance; withholding this type of body contact may communicate an uncaring or disinterested attitude.

In medicine, patients are constantly being physically touched by doctors, nurses, aides, and attendants. The most intimate body parts are manipulated by hand and instrument often in a painful and intrusive manner. The way in which the professional touches the patient can communicate hurry, harassment, disinterest, embarrassment, insecurity, incompetence; or concern, caring, reassurance, competence. A patient may rapidly lose confidence in the professional who tactually communicates inexperience in contrast to the more experienced hand.

Tactile communication within a group may be used by the leader as an intervention or to develop an analysis of the status of the group or its members. In the former, the leader may hold or touch a member who is experiencing difficulty or rejection as a gesture of comfort, support, or reassurance. In the latter, the leader-observer may use tactile communication to assess the feeling-tone (e.g., cohesiveness and closeness among members) of the group. A great deal of touching can be an indicator that a group is concerned and cares for its members, that it seeks to provide much support and reassurance. Little touching can indicate a lack of concern, a climate of impersonality or formality. Naturally any interpretations based on these observations must take into consideration a range of other factors in addition to touching per se: e.g., the setting, the culture, the sex of the participants, and so forth.

Proxemics

Proxemics involves the study of communication by and through the use of space. The early research on animals' defense of territory provided the impetus for parallel studies of human territoriality. In particular, a concern has been directed toward studying conversation distances that persons use for formal and informal interaction (Hall, 1959; 1963; Little, 1968). Research has suggested a cultural variation in this distance; in some cultures, for example, standing breath-to-breath for all conversations is considered appropriate. This often confuses the cultural alien who is used to having greater distance (e.g., 3 feet) between self and others. Violating this distance breaks the implicit shield some people carry around themselves, often creating unintended messages. For example, if 3 to 5 feet in distance is considered comfortable for a typical conversation in the United States, then whenever persons stand either closer or farther away, they are communicating something beyond the usual. Excessive closeness may communicate greater intimacy than is desired; distance may indicate a wish to break off the interaction by taking leave.

Sometimes group members move their chairs closely together as a mood of warmth and camaraderie takes over during a meeting. The keen observer of proxemics can determine much about the cohesiveness of a group by noting the arrangement of chairs during or after a meeting. Subgroup formation may likewise often be determined by simply noting which individuals spatially cluster together and how much distance separates them from other subgroups.

An intervention technique usefully employed in some types of groups actually builds upon proxemic communication. The technique involves placing a marker in the center of the room (e.g., a piece of paper or an X to mark the center). Members are asked to consider that center mark as being the ideal group member or the most ideal group they can imagine. Members are then asked to locate themselves around that marker, using their distance from it to indicate how closely they feel they approximate the ideal. After persons have arranged themselves, the leader then asks each to talk about why they located themselves as they did, how others feel about each person's location, and what steps would be needed to move each person closer in toward that ideal spot.

This technique often reveals a great deal about the group. For example, it can reveal subgroup formations as some members cluster themselves together and separated from others. It can reveal members who feel themselves separate from the group—some may actually locate themselves outside the meeting room or at the doorway. Proxemics can be a useful too to determine group members' feelings about the group or about their function within the group.

Compensation.   A principle of *compensation* has been noted by some analysts of proxemic behavior (Argyle & Dean, 1965; Patterson, 1968). When an individual stands too close for comfort, there is a tendency for the other person to compensate by averting the eyes, leaning backwards, or by presenting a side rather than a straight-on body orientation. On the other hand, when someone stands beyond the comfort range, compensation involves the other person's leaning forward and staring more directly into the other's eyes.

Immediacy Cues.   One investigator, Mehrabian (1971), has introduced the concept of immediacy cues to refer to a set of nonverbal, primarily proxemic (but including kinesic as well) information that communicates the *degree of liking or disliking that is involved in a relationship.* Immediacy cues involve distance, body orientation, and eye gaze. Thus, if a person stands at some distance from another, orients his or her body away from that person, and tends not to look at the other, the message of dislike or of impersonality may well be nonverbally communicated. Note that the person may not have consciously intended this message; nevertheless, the receiver picks up the message and may respond accordingly.

Impressions.   Many of our impressions of others are derived on the basis of their nonverbal behavior; their impressions of us are likewise influenced by our nonverbal as well as our verbal messages. Clearly, the observer of group process must become sensitive to members' nonverbal behavior in order to understand what is going on. For example, normative pressures may be communicated nonverbally; deviant members are rejected proxemically, for example, by other members locating themselves at some distance or refusing to interact with a more friendly, face-to-face body orientation.

Likewise, the observer may note that a member communicates her attitude proxemically, by the way in which she locates herself spatially in the group. A member may express anger, for example, by physcially separating herself from other group members. Or another may be communicating disinterest or boredom by leaning back or away from the rest of the group. The observer must be sensitive to this form of information, especially, for example, when a member's opinions have been criticized and he physically withdraws from further participation. The use of space communicates to the observer and others that person's feeling or rejection; he says *spatially* what he feels. This observation may motivate the observer-leader to intervene to help bring the member back into the group or to help him deal with his feelings of rejection.

The implications for the practicing health professional are critical. When we realize how much our impressions of patients and their impressions of us derives from nonverbal proxemic information, and in turn, how those impressions can seriously influence the success of our practice, we must reassess this mode of our communication. For example, the dying patient often first becomes aware of this prognosis when the nurses proxemically (and inadvertently) communicate it to them. Although they use reassuring words, their spatial separation and avoidance speaks to the patient much louder than anything they say verbally.

Status and Proxemics. Proxemic communication involves many complex interpersonal issues. Sommer's work (1969) has been especially instructive in showing how persons arrange the spatial features in a room or at a table in order to communicate something to others. For example, people who wish to be left alone may communicate this desire nonverbally by locating themselves at the end of a rectangular table; or they may place themselves squarely in the center, surrounded by territorial markers (e.g., coats, books, etc.) to communicate "this is my table and I don't want anyone else to sit nearby."

Power and status are likewise communicated spatially: sitting behind a large desk facing the patient and others from behind its protective barrier emphasizes formality of relationship between persons of differing power and status. Proxemic messages are used extensively in small groups. People who wish to adopt the leadership position within the group may literally situate themselves spatially so as to be at the group's center or at its spatial focal point.

Kinesics

Kinesic communication primarily involves a language of gestures, including movements of the body, limbs, the face, and especially the eyes. There has been an extensive array of research attempting to uncover the meanings of body language. There is much debate concerning whether or not persons universally express themselves kinesically in the same way, or if there are culture and situation-specific modes of kinesic communication. For example, is anger universally expressed by the same facial gestures or do these vary by culture? For the observer of group process, it is less important to resolve such an issue than to be able to recognize and become proficient in noting how others use their bodies and their eyes to communicate. Kinesic communication provides a rich source of information about persons' feelings and thoughts and about the kinds of relationships that emerge when two or more people interact.

Leakage. Paul Ekman's work has been especially enlightening regarding the importance of kinesic communication (Ekman, 1964; 1965a; b; Ekman & Friesan, 1969; 1974; Ekman, et al., 1972). One investigation suggested the principle of *nonverbal leakage*. Ekman believed that individuals are more in control of facial and head cues than bodily cues, and thus the body is more likely than the head to "leak" real feelings. To study this, Ekman filmed individuals who were intentionally being deceptive about their true feelings, trying to hide them from others. He showed these films to several groups, some of whom saw only the deceiver's head, others only the body, and still others the full person. Ekman's expectation that the body would show the true feelings better than the head was substantiated. People who had seen either the full individual or the body were more accurate in surmising that person's deception than were those who saw only the head. The implication for the practitioner is obvious; if we have reason to believe that people are intentionally trying to deceive us or even that they may be ignorant of their own real feelings, we can learn a great deal by attending to body gestures that "leak" these feelings.

MMEs. Additional research reported by Ekman demonstrated the importance of what he termed *micromomentary expressions* (MME). These refer to rather small movements of muscle groups in the face. Some of these movements are so tiny, in fact, that the typical viewer can discern them easily only when they have been filmed and the film is shown at a very slow speed. Yet there are some people who seem capable of noting these MMEs even during interaction, suggesting an important individual difference in the capability of perceiving nonverbal kinesic behavior. We return to this issue of individual differences shortly.

Attention to MMEs can offer the observer further information about the feelings and attitudes of others. A patient, for example, may verbally express little concern about a forthcoming surgical procedure; perhaps in our own eagerness to avoid dealing with his or her tension, we accept that person's verbal message at face value and probe no further. However, the keen observer may note the patient's more subtle gestures (i.e., MMEs) that inform us of anxiety and tension. Such practitioners are now better equipped to help the patient; they have recognized the tension expressed nonverbally and thus can work more effectively with the patient before surgery.

Eyes. Kinesics also involves movements of the hands and the eyes. The eyes are especially informative. Exline and his associates demonstrated how either excessive or too little eye contact between persons can be discomforting (see Exline, 1971). Some research showed, for example, how 0 percent or 100 percent eye contact was less comfortable than eye contact in the 50 percent range. Thus, people who stare relentlessly at others may inadvertently communicate in ways that cause them to be disliked or feared; their excessive eye contact may increase tension and aversion in others.

Other investigations have suggested that people seem to prefer more eye contact when the communication is positive and less when it is negative (e.g., Ellsworth & Carlsmith, 1968). The power implications of eye contact have also been demonstrated. Exline's work suggested a tendency for those low in power to look more at those in high power than vice versa. Furthermore, persons who are seeking to establish dominance in a relationship are thought to attempt to "capture" the other's gaze.

Once again, we can readily note the implications of these findings for the observer of group process as well as for the practitioner. Observers can use their assessment of eye contact within group interaction, for example, as one way of evaluating the power relationships that exist or are being sought: e.g., who tries to capture other's glances; who is looked at most frequently.

We have noticed in some of our own work with groups, for example, that certain members will frequently look at the leader. They seem forever trying to examine the leader as though to determine what he or she is thinking. One interpretation of this observation is that such members may be insecure and are seeking approval and direction from the person in authority. Of course, this is not the only interpretation possible, but it is one that warrants consideration and attempts to validate: e.g., "I've noticed that you frequently look at me. I'm not sure what this means or what you want, but I have the feeling that you are waiting for me to do something or to say something."

Leadership. Another substantial contribution to kinesic communication has been made by Birdwhistell (1952), who observed how leadership in a group of adolescent boys was communicated kinesically rather than verbally. An observer of the boys' verbal behavior would note little difference between the group's leader and other members with respect to initiating conversations or frequency of participation. However, group leaders were noted to be "kinesically more mature" than group members. They engaged in less fidgeting, less foot shuffling, fewer extraneous movements. Furthermore, posturally, they were especially good and attentive listeners: that is, their gestural language communicated interest in, concern for, and attention to others in their group. Their leadership was communicated primarily through their nonverbal, kinesic movements rather than by what they said or how frequently they said it.

Hands. Hand movements, in particular hand rubbing, has come under the scrutiny of another team of investigators concerned with kinesic behavior (Freedman, Blass, Rifkin, & Quitkin, 1973). That research demonstrated a fascinating link between hand movements and verbal behavior. Specifically, it was found that during periods in which the individual was covertly hostile and angry, hand movements peaked. During periods of direct, overt hostility, hand rubbing decreased and hand movements tended to be used more to emphasize the verbal hostility: e.g., the hands were used to punctuate the anger that was being overtly expressed verbally. The keen observer may be able to determine another's attitudes and feelings by watching their hand movements rather than depending solely on their verbal communication.

Paralinguistics

The final category of nonverbal communication involves paralinguistic behavior—verbalizations that are not, strictly speaking, words. These include intonations, pauses, pitch, intensity, the use of such sounds as "uh-huh," and so forth. Kasl and Mahl's research (1965) has demonstarted an important link between tension and the excessive use of "uh" and similar utterances. The trained practitioner can become sensitive to paralinguistic signs of tension or anxiety: e.g., the client's voice may crack, his or her pace may quicken, pauses may lengthen, intonation may flaten. The latter is especially informative about depression.

Paralinguistics provides the observer with a rich source of information about group feelings as well as individual feelings. An entire group may demonstrate boredom on the one hand or involvement or anxiety on the other through paralinguistic means. Long, rambling, and monotonously intoned conversations within the group, for example, might inform the leader that involvement and interest are low. This should motivate a search for possible reasons: e.g., perhaps group members are bored and disinterested because they are unclear about their purposes or goals, or because the task is one that was designed for them by the leader rather than the one that they agreed to do. Rapidly paced, quick bursts of conversation or conversation that is high-pitched and intense can indicate either excitement or anxiety in the group. Further observations of other kinds of verbal and nonverbal material are required to determine which of these is present: e.g., we are likely to affirm an interpretation of anxiety rather than joyful excitement if we also observe some members' physical withdrawal, hear and see rapid breathing, hear content that involves difficulties, tensions, and conflict.

INDIVIDUAL DIFFERENCES
IN NONVERBAL BEHAVIOR

As has been noted, there are cultural as well as individual differences in nonverbal behavior. Individual differences within the same general cultural group are especially important to understand. Ekman's research suggested that although some people appear to be more sensitive to MMEs than others, most people can be trained to develop sensitivity to microexpressions. A kind of intuitive "feeling" for the moods and feelings of others may reflect a high sensitivity. It is possible to train individuals to develop more empathy as they develop their abilities to observe and to be responsive to nonverbal communications.

Senders

Another type of critical individual difference pertains less to the receiver or observer of the nonverbal behavior than to the sender. Some important experimental research has demonstrated, for example, a rather striking difference between males and females in their abilities as senders of nonverbal messages (Buck, et al., 1974). Teams were composed with one person assigned the role of sender and the other the role of receiver (i.e., observer). Each sender was given some pictures to examine while the receiver observed the nonverbal, primarily facial responses to these pictures from an adjoining room. The receiver's task was simply to identify the picture that the sender was examining entirely on the basis of nonverbal facial cues. Teams with male senders did less well than teams with female senders. In other words, the ability to accurately read another person's nonverbal behavior, in this instance, appeared to be a function of individual variations in the ability to clearly send nonverbal messages, rather than a function of the training of the observer.

If we may generalize beyond these findings, the implication is that some persons provide us with less helpful nonverbal indicators of their feelings and attitudes than do others. Yet even here the data emphasize facial communication. The range of nonverbal cues we have noted is substantial; the observer may be able to determine ways in which poor facial senders communicate through other channels. At least, the trained observer-practitioner would not expect his or her male clients (or male group members) to be as helpful in their facial nonverbal indications as their female clients; thus the observer-practitioner would do well to become more attentive to other channels of nonverbal communication that may be informative for males.

VERBAL VS. NONVERBAL BEHAVIOR

According to Bateson and others, all communication contains two levels of message and meaning (see e.g., Ruesch & Bateson, 1951). The first involves the actual content of the message and is called the *communication*. The second, called the *metacommunication*, says something about the relationship that is involved between the persons who are interacting. Typically, the communication is conveyed verbally and the metacommunication is conveyed nonverbally. The concept of *double-bind* was developed to describe discrepancies between these two aspects (Bateson et al, 1956).

Double-Bind

A double-bind exists when the discrepancy between the communication and the metacommunication poses a dilemma for the receiver of the conflicting messages. Does the receiver respond to the communication or to the metacommunication? For example, a mother greets her institutionalized son. Verbally she says, "How good it is to see you again." This is the content aspect of her message and is positive in tone. Nonverbally, however, her body stiffens, her hands become rigid, and she holds him at some distance from herself. This is the metacommunicational aspect; it says that she is not eager to be there seeing him. To which message does the boy respond—the positive verbal communication or the rejecting metacommunication? He is said to be caught in a double-bind. If he follows the metacommunication and acts as though she were rejecting, she can counter by claiming she meant what she said verbally; however, if he follows the verbal message, he may respond inappropriately to her real feelings of rejection.

Observers of group interaction can note many instances of the double-bind as well as other discrepancies between communication and metacommunication. They will see, for example, persons verbally communicating one way to their group, while nonverbally expressing an opposing message. The dilemma for the group is to clarify which meaning they should respond to. Senders, of course, may not be aware of their double messages and so will remain puzzled about why people respond to them as they do.

Does Ruth really mean "No, I don't want to take over the leadership" when she utters these words, or do we respond to her metacommunication of apparent eagerness? Does Betty really not want to talk or is she really eager to express her opinions? Suppose someone says to her, "Betty, I've noticed that you have been silent during most of this discussion. Is there anything you would care to tell us about this issue?" She smiles, her eyes brighten noticeably, she leans forward in her chair, shuffles her feet, and says, "No, I'm happy just remaining quiet and watching you all discuss the project." Should the questioner then sit back and accept the verbal communication, or decide that she really means what the *metacommunication* reveals—namely that she would like to talk but needs a little more pushing, an invitation to enter into the discussion? If she is taken at her word and isn't pushed a little, she might feel rejected. If she is encouraged to talk, she may provide a useful contribution.

Observers of family interaction often note a similar dilemma, as we see in this example:

> Ralph receives a call at work from Roger, an old family friend. Roger is in town for only one day; without consulting his wife, Ralph invites Roger over for dinner. He then calls up his wife, Sue, to tell her to expect a third for dinner. She says she is eager to see the old family friend, and excitedly prepares the dinner. Later that evening, Ralph and Sue get involved in a rather nasty argument over Roger's coming to dinner. The puzzling fact about their communication is that they are basically in agreement; their argument seems to make little sense. Both agree that it was a great idea to have Roger over for dinner; both were pleased to see him again. But by taking the initiative to invite Roger over for dinner without first consulting his wife, Ralph has declared something about the power relationship between himself and Sue. Their battle is over the power each has in decision making, a metacommunicational issue. (From Watzlawick, Beavin & Jackson, 1967).

This case is more complex than the simpler double-bind example (e.g., mother and son) or the typical cases involving a discrepancy between what the person says verbally and what she or he says nonverbally (e.g., Ruth or Betty in the group). In this case, we must attend to a complex set of communications between the husband and the wife rather than one or two simple statements. In many different ways, each tells the other how pleased they are to have Roger over, how good it is to see him again, how much they both like him, and so forth. Yet in many different ways, each also implies that it was wrong (from the wife's perspective) or right (from the husband's) for Ralph to have made the decision without consulting Sue. The analysis of this case, therefore, requires a consideration of what are ostensibly paragraphs and pages of interaction rather than a single, isolated message. The point, however, remains the same: there are two discrepant levels of meaning.

In general terms, this case highlights a common aspect of group interaction. People often become involved in heated arguments even while they are in apparent agreement over issues of content. Members may be in apparent agreement over the content of a proposed decision, but cannot actually make and act upon it. They get wrapped up in argumentation and become immobilized. Why? Examine the meta-communicational messages that are involved. These messages often say something about the power and authority relationships that exist and that lead members to resist acting upon decisions that imply, "I have less power than you, because you first suggested the idea."

Hidden Agenda. The metacommunications mentioned above make up much of a group's *hidden agenda,* an agenda that must be adequately dealt with before the group's more formally stated agenda can be satisfactorily negotiated. Recall the discussion in Chapter 5. A hidden agenda is related to socioemotional issues—those that have to do with maintaining internal order and harmony. As we previously noted, unless these matters are resolved, groups will flounder helplessly and ineffectively; the same issues will recur again and again; no decisions or actions will be accomplished, and the group's work will never get done.

The observer can learn to be sensitive to the hidden agendas that are usually conveyed via metacommunication: i.e., to the issues of member–member relationships that are implied even when the members agree about the actual content of their discussion. It is helpful to focus members' attention on their agreements in content in order to clarify for them that the issue lies elsewhere, in their hidden agenda.

"AS-IF" APPROACHES TO ASSESSMENT

To act "as-if" is to take another person's role and attempt to see and experience through his or her eyes. It is by no means an easy thing to do; yet it is an important assessment technique. There are really two related as-if techniques. The first involves the use of actual role-playing within groups in order to better evaluate and understand some aspect of group process. The second asks observers to put themselves figuratively into the situation by empathizing with the persons involved, thereby to gain a better appreciation of what is going on in the group. Let us briefly examine each of these as-if approaches in turn.

Role-Playing

Role-playing techniques can provide a useful approach to understanding. They involve creating a situation that portrays some issue, problem, or event within the group. An example of role-playing will illustrate this point.

The group contains eight persons, six of whom have been meeting together for several weeks. Two new members will be added to an existing group of six. The leader anticipates that the introduction of the new members will pose an issue that should be dealt with immediately by the group rather than left alone, perhaps to emerge later to interfere with the group's functioning. The leader feels that an issue exists both for the continuing members, who now have to learn about these new people and how to relate to them, and for the two strangers, who must figure out their place in the group. She expects, for example, that the new members will feel isolated from the others, that they may be reluctant to express themselves openly and to participate actively in the group. It is also likely that the continuing members will resent these outsiders and ignore them or put on a show for them: "see how we do things in our group." The leader has decided to confront the new/old issue head on through role-playing. The leader creates a role-playing situation in which an old member portrays a new member and a new member portrays the old. In other words, she creates a *role reversal* so that individuals can gain a better appreciation of the meanings of being "new" and "old" in this group. After the role-playing, a discussion is held in order to explore the feelings and experiences that emerged. Toward the end of the session and at the next meeting, all members express feeling much better about their group than before the role-playing. The new members feel themselves to be an active part of the group; simply having participated in a role-playing exercise has helped integrate them better. Likewise, old members, sensitized to the feelings of being new, are more inclined to incorporate the new persons into their group.

In the example, the leader anticipated an issue and used a role-playing technique, role reversal, to focus attention on this issue and to provide material for group discussion and analysis. In many cases, issues emerge during the course of group interactions that readily lend themselves to some form of role-playing. For example, a conflict between different opinions may be helpfully clarified by asking the participants to role-play the opposing sides, thereby giving everyone a better view of both opinions.

Role-playing need not involve role reversals. The use of role-playing in training proves especially helpful in giving trainees a sense of the kinds of job-related issues they are likely to meet; it gives them and their associates an opportunity to work through these issues in a more concrete way rather than or in addition to discussing them in more general, abstract terms. For example, the nurse who must deal with a dying patient can be helped by role-playing the situation. One person plays the patient while others take on roles as members of the family.

The role-playing permits issues to emerge that might not otherwise be confronted except in the real situation. While acting out this situation, the nurse may discover that she tends to avoid talking about the issue with the patient or his family; she may look to the side, avert her gaze, and in other ways communicate her troubles in confronting death. Role-playing allows these aspects of her behavior to come directly to light so they can be dealt with; thus she becomes better prepared to deal with the actual situation when she encounters it.

Role-playing techniques are useful in two aspects of the assessment process: for discovery and for working through issues that have been uncovered. In the example, by role-playing, the nurse is helped to discover her attitudes toward death and dying by seeing these attitudes emerge in her own behavior. In addition to this discovery, role-playing permits her to *work through* her attitudes. She is allowed to try out alternative ways of relating to the patient and his family and to experiment with ways of coping with a potentially difficult situation.

Empathy

The second type of as-if approach involves the process of *empathy*. Basically, this requires that the observer-practitioner figuratively place him- or herself in the shoes of someone else—this way the individual must ask *"How would I feel if I were that person in these circumstances?"*

A team of health professionals has been meeting to discuss and evaluate the treatment plans for selected cancer patients. An issue emerges between two members who have known one another outside the group and who have formed rather negative feelings that interfere with their functioning within the group. It becomes obvious to everyone that these two may never agree on any proposal that is made because they use all proposals as a vehicle for continuing their outside battle. As a result, the whole group is bogged down and unable to make progress. Thus, it has become imperative to deal with the issue so that the group can function again. But one member of the arguing pair, Janice, refuses to talk about the outside issue. The group leader decides to employ a version of the as-if technique. She figuratively places herself in Janice's shoes, seeking to experience the situation as though she were Janice. The group leader then says, "If I were you, Janice, I would really be angry and upset right now. How do you feel?" This technique, repeated on several different occasions, helps Janice feel that she has an understanding ally; thus she begins to feel freer to begin to deal with her own feelings. Soon, the group is able to get back to its major task issues.

In the example, the leader acts as if she *is* the other person and speaks for her, expressing what Janice might feel or want to say but is hesitant to say. Of course, it is possible for the leader to make incorrect assessments or an assessment that is premature and thus is not useful. In this case, the "problem" person will usually simply reject the leader's as-if statements. In the illustration, however, the leader's assessment helped lead the group past this block to its continued progress.

Empathy can be used in groups by either the leader or the members; it can be used in groups of colleagues and of patients. By actively attempting to gain the other person's perspective, to see and to experience the situation from the other side, the health professional is able to make a better assessment of the situation and to intervene in a helpful manner.

Let us examine one further example. A member of the team is dealing with a 44-year-old woman who is facing surgery for breast cancer. By placing herself in that woman's situation, the professional can ask herself: "How would I feel if I were 44, attractive, and facing the possible loss of my breast tomorrow? What kinds of things would I be worried about? I would worry about my husband and how he might feel toward me. I would worry about what else might be found once I was cut open. I would be frightened." Seeing and experiencing from the patient's perspective, as if one is the patient, can be invaluable in the health professional's understanding and intervention.

A Caution.   Using oneself as the key assessment tool can involve pitfalls. We too often project ourselves and our own biases onto the other rather than experiencing the situation in that person's terms. The risk, then, is that we might not be acting or experiencing as if we were the other person but rather as we might do or feel. Caution is required. However, in many situations, the feelings are sufficiently common and shared that we can be relatively secure in trying to view the situation through the eyes of another.

OBSERVING VERBAL BEHAVIOR

In observing people's verbal communications, we confront a rich and variable source of material. We can focus on the *content* of what is said, noting, for example, what kinds of questions are asked, what theme or issue are people talking about. And we can focus on the *form* or the ways in which things are expressed—for example, who asks questions and who gives answers? In this latter case, we are not really attending to what is said but rather to its form: that is, it is not the content that we examine, but rather the expression of that content. While it is possible to separate content from form, we are usually interested in observing both features of verbal behavior. Furthermore, we must realize that the content of a verbal communication may be conveyed directly (e.g., "Shut up!"), somewhat indirectly (e.g., "I think it is a bit noisy in here") or very indirectly (e.g., "I went to a film the other night and had great difficulty in hearing, there were so many kids around just talking among themselves"). Let us look at an informative example that illustrates several of these points.

> When the family members gather together with the psychologist and social worker to discuss Mrs. Aberle's pending breast surgery, the psychologist says: "I think it will be helpful if we examine our feelings about the upcoming surgery and use this occasion to ask any questions that you may have". This is what he observes in response:

Observations of Verbal Behavior

1. Mr. Aberle begins to talk about the last time he went to the hospital, noting that it was to the ER for what turned out to be a relatively minor matter.
2. Mrs. Aberle's mother, who lives in the Aberle household, notes that her own health is poor and that she gets anxious whenever she has to go to the hospital: "I just don't trust those doctors."
3. Rob, the 14-year-old son, mentions the cold symptoms he's been having.
4. Gail, the 16-year-old daughter, comments on Rob's never being able to take proper care of himself and how she always has to mother him.
5. Mr. Aberle comments again about his own experiences with doctors and hospitals, noting how things always turn out to be worse in anticipation than in realization.
6. Gwen says to Mr. Aberle, "You just don't understand, do you! I'm frankly worried about it."

The content of much of this family's remarks focuses on each person's experience with illness and with doctors. Mr. Aberle seems to deny that there is really anything to worry about, almost reassuring himself. The patient's mother directly and openly expresses her anxiety about her daughter's operation and expresses the same doubts that her daughter probably also feels. The son, Rob, seems to find it easier to focus on his own problems rather than openly confronting his mother's pending surgery. Gail, in turn, seems to be expressing her anxiety about the new role she will have to take on (mother) as her mother is forced to withdraw from these functions for a while. She might also be expected to be anxious about the implications of breast surgery for herself. The content, therefore, can be very revealing about how each member of this family relates to Mrs. Aberle's surgery and its special meaning to them.

Note that the focus is not simply on the content as such, but on the verbal content as an answer (direct or indirect) to the question, "How do you each feel about the surgery?" Thus, when Mr. Aberle's response is to relate his own recent hospital visit that turned out to be something relatively minor ("I'm not worried—after all it must be minor just like my own experience"), the acute observer will realize that this denial of the seriousness of the procedure is an issue that will have to be dealt with.

The form of the verbal communication in the example above suggests the following: (1) Everyone answers the psychologist's question by personalizing it; that is, all relate one of their own experiences that is intended to carry or convey their feelings in a less direct manner. (2) There is disagreement within the family regarding the seriousness of the surgery. In particular, we note the difference between Mr. Aberle and his mother-in-law. We might even detect some hostility generating between them as she tries to convince everyone of the seriousness of the operation and the problems involved and as he tries to convince everyone that it is not a major matter. (3) All family members except the patient's mother use an indirect mode of expression. She is fairly direct in expressing her concerns.

SOCIOLINGUISTICS

It would take us too far beyond the interests of the introductory level to do more than briefly mention the emerging field of sociolinguistics (e.g., Ervin-Tripp, 1969; Gumperz & Hymes, 1972); we have touched on aspects of this approach to understanding verbal behavior in an earlier example involving forms of address (Chapter 3). To oversimplify, the observer uses the structural features of language behavior in order to understand the social relationships that exist within groups.

We noted previously, for example, how the forms of address used reflect the degree of formality or informality that is involved within a group as well as the nature of the authority relationship that exists. In a similar manner, the observer can note other features of language and from these learn still more about group processes.

Language Codes

Investigators have demonstrated that most of us are facile in using several different language codes in our everyday conversations (e.g., Bernstein, 1971, 1973; Hymes, 1964). For example, we can use a relatively formal code when giving a lecture or speaking in a formal gathering; yet with our friends, we drop some of the formality and switch to more colloquial language forms. Research has shown that by observing just the language code that is used within a group, it is possible to make inferences about the nature of the relationships within that group and about the social status of the members. One investigator (Labov, 1966; 1972) demonstrated the "r-less" quality of street language (e.g., the words, "four," "door," "car" and so forth lose their "r" sound) in New York in contrast to the return of "r" when the same persons are speaking formally or trying to communicate the impression of higher status.

To take another example, one team of investigators (Blom & Gumperz, 1972) noted that when engaged in trading, members of a Norwegian town spoke one language form (standard Norwegian) but switched to another (a local dialect) when dealing with personal matters. That is, they had one language code for business and another for less formal relationships. Clearly, an observer sensitive to these features of language behavior could learn a great deal about a group simply by noting the forms used in communications.

The issue of language code is especially relevant to the health professional in his or her work with patients and with the public (e.g., in community settings, with patient groups, and so forth). It is not unusual, for example, for medical professionals to communicate in the technical language of their field and in so doing completely confuse or bypass the patient who is equipped to understand a far less technical code.

> In a sexuality group, the nurse speaks about coitus, the clitoris, vaginal discharge, and so forth, assuming that these terms communicate her points to the public. The audience leaves without asking questions that

might reveal their failure to understand and her failure to communicate. They may feel that they now have learned something and she may feel that she has taught something. And yet no real educational process has occurred.

In a hospital, the nurse or the nurse's aide is giving the patient a bath. She hands the washrag to the patient, saying, "Now you finish your bath— I'll be back in a few minutes." When she returns, she notes that the patient has washed his hair, his face and his hands, but has not washed the genital area, which is what she intended him to do when she left the room. Although her language was not technical as such, it was part of a language code that communicates only to members of the in-group and not to the patient group for whom it is intended.

A sensitivity to and awareness of differences between the language codes of different groups is essential for the health professional. In these cases, the codes are not simply informative about the nature of the relationship that is involved (e.g., whether it involves friends or is more impersonal), but rather gets to the very heart of professional-patient communication. Professionals must become facile in determining the terms of language usage that are employed among the patient groups they are working with; they must then develop a facility in using those codes in order to communicate and inform.

Language and Thought

Some investigators (e.g., Bernstein, 1971; 1973) have proposed the important hypothesis that language usage and cognitive functioning— that is, the way people think and respond to one another—are intimately linked. Specifically, it has been suggested that some language codes, termed restricted, make it difficult to engage in the more subtle aspects of conversation; they constrain people to act more directly and physically rather than using words to analyze and describe a feeling, a situation, or even a symptom. Some individuals lack the words and concepts to describe inner bodily events or to make coherent sense out of things that have happened. Although there is some evidence that there is a social-class factor at work in these matters—some class-based language codes make it more difficult and other codes make it easier to verbally express complex and subtle ideas—more than social class seems to be involved. For the observer of verbal behavior, however, there is a rich territory of material open to systematic observation and analysis.

For the practitioner, of course, these kinds of difference in language codes and ability to provide rich descriptions of symptoms, for example, suggest the importance of developing alternative ways to obtain necessary information from patients. They also suggest that patients may need help in learning the terms and concepts that make the kinds of differentiations which their everyday language does not permit, but which the health professional feels is critical for their practice.

An Example: The Pelvic Exam. Observing how others speak, the forms they use, the manner by which verbal descriptions are generated, what specific terms are employed, can be informative to the trained observer, as is shown in the following example:

> Dr. Joan Emerson (Ph.D.) observed a number of pelvic examinations, noting among other things how the language used by the doctors and the nurses maintained the situation as a medical one rather than as a situation having more directly sexual meanings. She noted, for example, how "medical talk" helped to sustain the setting as nonsexual, whereas the intrusion of nonmedical talk threatened to make the setting inappropriately sexual. The staff used medical terms that help depersonalize the situation; formal terms rather than colloquial terms were used for body parts. Doctors talked about *the* vagina rather than *your* vagina, thereby making it even more impersonal. Instructions to the patient likewise were couched in a language that refuted any possible sexual imagery. Instead of the doctor asking the patient to "spread your legs," with its potential sexual connotations, "Let your knees fall apart" was frequently used. Emerson noted how patients' own language usage sought to minimize the personal quality of the exam; they too referred to pains "down there" or "down below." (From Emerson, 1975)

The trained observer is able to see how the language forms that are used in interaction help shape and sustain the meanings that develop. It is possible to learn a great deal, therefore, by taking careful note of how others express themselves, what address forms they use, what language codes they select, and what terms they employ to describe and to refer to themselves and others.

THE BALES SYSTEM

One of the best-known systems available for systematically analyzing verbal interaction within groups was proposed several years ago by R.F. Bales (1950a,b; 1970). He provides categories that involve the broader aspects of group interaction, encompassing many different kinds of content. Furthermore, although he emphasized the analysis of verbal behavior, he believes the observer should use both verbal and nonverbal cues to make a decision about the category to which a particular utterance should be assigned.

Bales developed his system for observing and recording communication based on his theory regarding the two major areas of concern to all groups: *task issues* and *socioemotional or maintenance issues.* We considered these in Chapter 2. Bales reasoned that communication could be primarily concerned with either task matters or maintenance issues. He developed a scheme that distinguished between these two major categories. Communication in the socioemotional or maintenance area, he believed, could be generally positive or generally negative; further, a distinction could be made within the task area as well. Bales therefore sought to distinguish between communications that *give out* material to others and those that *ask for* material from others. With these several distinctions in mind, Bales developed a twelve-category system for observing and recording communication within groups.

I. Communication Involving Task Issues

A. Giving or Sending to Others

1. Gives Suggestion: involves taking some lead and direction in task matters, including focusing the group's attention on a problem, organizing the group, developing an agenda, and so forth.

2. Gives Opinion: involves serious evaluation and analysis or commentary on the task, including reasoning, judgment, elaboration, diagnosis, etc.

3. Gives Orientation: involves providing information and clarification of points and issues, helping to orient the group to its task, conveying knowledge relevant to dealing with the task.

B. Asking for or Receiving Material From Others

4. Asks for Suggestion: involves a concern that is parallel to category #1; emphasizes needing some direction, requesting an agenda, turning the initiative over to another, etc.

5. Asks for   parallels category #2; seeks to elicit or to
   Opinion: encourage reactions on the part of oth-
                     ers; tries to elicit opinions from others
                     on various items and issues that come
                     before the group.

6. Asks for   parallels category #3; involves seeking
   Orientation: factual type information or clarification
                     of still confusing matters.

II. Communications Involving Maintenance Issues

A. Emotionally Positive Expressions

7. Shows Solidarity: involves acting in a generally supportive
                     and friendly way, helpful to others, car-
                     ing of others, expressing harmony and
                     unity.

8. Shows Tension   involves acts that joke, laugh, or dram-
   Release: atize in such a way as to help break ten-
                     sion or produce a sense of elation.

9. Agrees: involves acceptance, concurrence, com-
                     pliance with others, understanding oth-
                     ers, being receptive and interested.

B. Emotionally Negative Expressions

10. Disagrees: withholds help from others; passively
                     rejects others; can also include showing
                     disbelief in others' comments or ideas;
                     nonresponsive.

11. Shows Tension: symptoms of anxiety and tension, in-
                     cluding inappropriate laughter, exces-
                     sive hesitation, tremor, blocking in
                     speech; may also involve withdrawal
                     and hanging back from issues; showing
                     fear or apprehension.

12. Shows   involves unfriendly acts, acts that de-
   Antagonism: flate others, that are defensive, that
                     seem presumptuous or condescending;
                     also includes acts that indicate alien-
                     ation from others, boredom, noncaring,
                     lack of concern.

To use Bales' system, we should not only learn the meaning of each category; we also must learn to record communications on a who-to-whom matrix over time. Thus, to use this scheme in a systematic manner, we would indicate

—WHO: which group member is speaking?
—SAYS WHAT: into which of the twelve categories is the utterance to be located?
—TO WHOM: which member receives the message, or is it directed to the group in general?
—WHEN: when in the sequence of the meeting is the comment made?

Uses

Admittedly, it is likely that only a researcher interested in obtaining a complete record of a group's communication patterns would use the Bales method in the manner indicated. The results of such work, however, can be rather striking. They would reveal a literal structure to the communication within a group, an outline of who contributes the most to group task and maintenance functions—e.g., who, though speaking a great deal, seems to contribute little; who is relatively antagonistic; who responds to whom; and so on. The time-sequencing analysis permits the investigator to discover developmental trends in the life of the group. We will return to some of these matters in Chapter 10.

If it is primarily the researcher who will use a scheme such as that of Bales in the systematic manner he suggests, then what use is such an approach to the health professional who simply wants to evaluate the status of a group? In our view, even though one might not use the Bales system (or some similar system) in precisely the way proposed, it does provide a way of systematically observing and thinking about interaction and communication within groups. It has been our experience that those who train themselves to use these categories become better observers of group interaction. They become sensitized to aspects of communication that the more casual observer tends to overlook. Thus, even though we might not be as systematic or complete as the researcher in our use of Bales system, efforts to practice observing interaction with this system will help increase our sensitivity to and awareness of communication within a group.

SUMMARY AND CONCLUSIONS

A convenient way of summarizing the complex interrelationship of verbal and nonverbal materials that are used in the assessment of group and individual process is represented in Table 9–1. This table provides a model that organizes the material introduced in this chapter (and several other chapters we have considered—e.g., chapters on theory) so that it can be used for purposes of assessment.

Several case examples using the material summarized in this chapter, as presented in Table 9-1, are presented for the reader's convenience in applying the principles of the assessment process.

Table 9–1. The Assessment Process

I.	Perception:	What do I see?	Attention to nonverbal behaviors
		What do I hear?	Attention to nonverbal and verbal behaviors
II.	Affect-Empathy:	How do I feel?	Attention to empathy; place self in the other's situation in order to better appreciate and understand his/her concerns
III.	Cognition:	What does it mean?	Development of hunches and tentative interpretations of the meaning of the observed behaviors; includes the ongoing examination of additional material that confirms or refutes hunches
IV.	Validation:	Is my assessment correct?	Involves testing the assessment: e.g., by asking questions; waiting to gather additional material; checking with others' assessments
V.	Intervention:	How shall I respond?	Involves making a decision based on the assessment regarding what actions to take: e.g., to intervene in a supportive way; to probe and question further, etc.

Case #1

The patient, Mrs. Percell, is a 44-year-old woman who has been hospitalized for a breast biopsy. You are talking with her before the full procedure. You are aware that she has had several previous contacts with medical personnel and so is assumed to be relatively well-informed about what will take place and its implications.

Perception.   You see Mrs. Percell sitting across from you, clenching her hands, rubbing them together frequently. She appears restless and moves about in her chair. She seems unable to sit still. Her legs, in particular, move. Her face muscles, especially around her lips, are tightened. Her speech is rapid; vocal pitch is high. Occasionally her voice cracks, at which moments she laughs nervously and then covers her mouth with her fingers. The content of her talk involves questions about her pending surgical procedure. This procedure has already been explained to her several times, yet she continues to focus her questions around its details. You notice that she frequently repeats the same question even after you have given what you think is a satisfactory answer.

Affect-Empathy.   Ask yourself how you would feel in her situation: you are 44, still young and fairly attractive. You know that you are awaiting a procedure that might result in the loss of one breast; you also know that even more than that can be involved. Frankly, you are frightened and worried about how you will look afterwards and who you will be to your husband, children, friends.

Cognition.   You can interpret the various observations as meaning that Mrs. Percell is anxious and is concerned about several issues pertaining to the impact of the procedure on her life. You can sense that these are the real matters that she needs to discuss with someone rather than the minor details that most of her questions seem to center on.

Validation.   You directly ask Mrs. Percell if she would find it helpful to talk over with you some of the implications of the biopsy for her and her life.

Intervention.   In part, your effort to validate your interpretation is the first step in intervention. You are not only asking her to check out and validate or refute your interpretation; in asking, you are indicating to her that you are sensitive to, aware of, and concerned about her feelings at this time. You are really inviting her to talk things over with you. You can then continue your intervention by suggesting, for example, that it must be a very frightening experience and that she might like to discuss that aspect with you. You could inquire about her husband: Has she talked things over with him yet? What was his reaction? How does she feel about his response to her? What concerns does she have about him? What other concerns and worries does she have?

Case #2

You are dealing with male post-coronary patients whose group you organized to help discuss and deal with issues of daily living. They eagerly signed up to attend several workshops under your direction; you assumed that their eagerness was motivated by their many questions and concerns that had not been resolved by other medical personnel with whom they had had contact.

Perception. You note that several of the men are restless, moving about in their chairs. Several look up toward the ceiling; a few gaze intently out the window. One or two open their mouth and take in a deep breath as though they are preparing to speak, but then say nothing. There are frequent silences, broken on occasion by desultory conversation. The voice quality of those who speak is very soft and hesitant. You are impressed by their tendency almost to speak in a whisper as if to save energy and avoid strain. The content of their talk tends to wander about; there are a few jokes made about sports and an occasional hint about something vaguely sexual. A couple briefly mention their jobs; and one member mentions something about being a man, but this is quickly dropped, replaced by a joke—and then silence.

Affect-Empathy. You realize that most of these men are in their late 40s to early 50s. They still have family concerns, children in college to support, large mortgage payments, jobs that are threatened by a tight job market. Place yourself in their situation and ask how you would feel if you were in their position. What kinds of concerns would you have? You would feel anxious about being able to function as you did before. Could you really keep your job and support your family? And if you couldn't, then what kind of a man would you be? And what about your sex life? Can you continue as before or must that too come to an end? And if you can't keep a job and can't keep active sexually, then who are you? Is life still worth living?

Cognition.   You would interpret the various indicators as suggesting that most of the members of the group are anxious, but perhaps not yet clear about just what all their concerns are. Perhaps they are even a bit embarrassed about mentioning what they might consider to be private and personal matters of jobs and sex, and so they engage in rather indirect and desultory conversation.

Validation.   Check your interpretation by saying something such as the following to the entire group: "I've noticed that we seem to have trouble getting started, trouble in talking about what some of our real concerns are. I wonder if people here are somewhat embarrassed to talk about what most worries them now? I realize that it may be difficult, but I wonder—are people here anxious about the effects of their coronary on their ability to continue their job, to continue maintaining a family, to continue their usual sexual activities? Maybe these are some of the things we should try and talk about."

Intervention.   In validating your hunch, you have already begun to intervene in the process of this group. It is important from this point on that you as a health professional be continually attentive to specific persons in the group and their modes of expression so that you can make it easy for each member to air his concerns and share with others.

10

Concepts and Types
of Leadership

"Leaders are born, not made." "Either you have what it takes to be a leader or you don't; there's no in between." "He's good at taking orders, but I'd never want him to lead the group." "She's a natural leader; there's nothing more she needs to learn about leadership." "Hell, it makes no difference who you're leading—they all need the same strong direction." "My best groups are those in which I don't do anything; they take the lead and it works fine."

*L*eadership has fascinated people since the beginnings of society. Who shall lead and who shall follow has often been of greater importance than where shall we go. Aristotle subscribed to the "great man" theory contained in several of our opening statements: that leaders are born, not made. Early studies located leadership in the personality of the leader. Numerous investigations were designed to determine those critical traits of personality and character that would help identify the leader (e.g., see Bass, 1960; Stogdill, 1948 for summaries). Not surprisingly, a substantial list of traits did emerge, but so too did several important counter-examples:

Leaders tend to be bigger and heavier than followers (Adolph Hitler?); stronger and healthier (Julius Caesar?); handsome and physically more attractive (Abraham Lincoln?); more aggressive and domineering (Mohandas Gandhi?); psychologically well adjusted (Nero?); more intelligent (please provide your own counter-example). In 1972 a political pundit pointed out that Americans prefer taller persons as president and that in every presidential election up until that time the taller of the two candidates had been elected. He predicted therefore, that George McGovern would handily defeat Richard Nixon. (Raven & Rubin, 1976, p. 372).

It may be, then, that leaders are made and not born.

Leadership and the Situation

As we think more critically about leadership, even our common sense directs us toward several different factors that go into leadership: personality and character, situation, task, and members. When the situation, members, and type of task are held fairly constant, certain personality traits emerge to describe group leaders. For example, dominance and assertiveness have been found to characterize the leaders of all-male groups in military-type contexts performing fairly routine problem-solving tasks. A change in personnel, setting, or task, however, reveals a different set of leadership traits. The person who can lead one type of group facing one type of task may not be the best to lead a different group facing a different task: e.g., Nurse Armstrong may be good in leading a group composed primarily of other nurses discussing a treatment plan, but may not be capable of leading a group of various other health professionals engaged in developing a proposal for a community-wide health care program.

What is Meant by Leadership?

To what are we referring when we talk about "leadership" and "leaders"? There are several possibilities (see Gibb, 1969):

1. One person who has been assigned the office or position of leader. This is often referred to as *headship* in order to distinguish between the formally appointed group leader and persons who informally take on group leadership.
2. Several persons who serve leadership functions, who act in those ways necessary for the group to work effectively toward its goals.
3. A person who is the central focus for the group, around whom the group forms and whose presence is necessary for the group's continuation and cohesiveness.
4. A person who is the most influential, who has the most power or the greatest ability to affect and alter the behavior of others.

Each of these describes an aspect of leadership. It is generally agreed that the most fruitful approach to the study of leadership is one ses on leadership functions rather than on a specific person as ~~artwright~~ & Zander, 1968; Gibb, 1969). The questions of lead- ~~ship~~ are thereby directed toward understanding the nature of these ~~func~~tions and their distribution within a group: e.g., does one person al~~w~~ays serve a particular function or is there a more equal distribution of functions across the membership? By focusing our attention on leadership functions, we also increase our sensitivity to the kinds of skills and knowledge that *all* people are able to bring to the group. Many individuals can and do serve leadership functions even though they may not have been formally appointed to such a position or have the title of group leader. Thus, by considering leadership as referring to *functions* rather than to persons, we can examine who serves those functions and how those functions are served within any particular group. We will note that at times the formally appointed group leader will serve many of the necessary functions; however, we will also note those times at which members come forward and serve necessary leadership functions.

Leadership Functions. What is meant by "leadership functions"? The list of leadership functions is extensive but usually includes the following (see Lippitt, 1961):

1. Helping the group decide on its purposes and goals.
2. Helping the group focus on its own process of working together so that it may become more effective rather than becoming trapped by faulty ways of problem solving and decision making.
3. Helping the group become aware of its own resources and how best to use them.
4. Helping the group evaluate its progress and development.
5. Helping the group to be open to new and different ideas without becoming immobilized by conflict.
6. Helping the group learn from its failures and frustrations as well as from its successes.

In talking about leadership functions, we are talking about actions and behaviors that any group member may carry out. Successful groups require that these functions be dealt with. No one person, however, need handle all of them. In fact, it is unlikely that a single person will be capable of effectively handling the multiplicity of functions that are necessary for the group to work well. Therefore, function #3 becomes important in most groups. The designated leader must work to utilize the resources and abilities of other members in order to handle the functions that he or she cannot personally manage.

Effective Leadership. Our analysis suggests that when we talk about leadership we are really referring to leadership functions. In this view, the skills of leadership involve the ability to get others to participate in leadership functions rather than in taking on the entire burden oneself. Leadership involves the effective utilization of a group's total resources; although one person may be designated group leader, effective resource utilization means that all members serve important leadership functions.

LEADERSHIP AS THE FACILITATION OF ASSETS OVER LIABILITIES

When a group comes together to work on a task or solve a problem, there are certain potential *assets* and certain potential *liabilities* that can develop (Maier, 1970). Let us briefly review some of these potential assets and liabilities.

ASSET: Since a group is composed of several individuals, there is often a wide and diverse range of ideas and information that can be called upon to solve a problem, make a decision, or get a job completed.

LIABILITY: Even though diversity exists, there are social pressures in all groups; members want to be accepted by others in their group. Often, the price of this acceptance is the avoidance of disagreements. Thus, diversity is silenced as members hope to gain acceptance by concealing rather than expressing their differences.

ASSET: Most solutions to issues and problems require their acceptance by members before they can be implemented. When members participate actively in their group, they are likely to accept the decisions that have been made. Furthermore, because decisions must be communicated from the decision makers to those who will implement them, the involvement of the latter with the former can help minimize distortion and faulty communication.

LIABILITY: Not everyone participates equally in the work of a group. Dominant members or a dominant leader may persuade others to adopt a solution that they really do not accept or agree with. Thus, when it comes time for them to implement the decision, they drag their feet or do it poorly. Furthermore, communications among members within a group can be distorted as members try to gain personal acceptance from others, to look good, and so forth.

Now that we have a sense of some of the possible assets and liabilities that stem from group work, let us examine the way in which a leader can influence whether a particular item will be an asset or a liability.

Diversity

The diversity of opinion, fact, and perspective that characterizes groups can be an asset if this diversity is brought to bear on problem solving; it can be a liability, however, if conflict and hard feelings develop among group members. A leader can try to reduce the expression of the diversity among members and thereby minimize conflict; yet the cost of doing this is to minimize the full utilization of the resources that diversity offers. And so, a leader can try to implement disagreement.

Certain leadership behaviors are helpful in creating a climate within which disagreement can be generated without running the risk of hard feelings and excessive, destructive conflict (see Maier, 1970):

1. The leader is open to perceiving disagreements rather than denying their presence.
2. The leader adopts a permissive attitude, one that allows members to express diverse opinions without fear of ridicule or rejection.
3. The leader helps the group to delay rushing into a decision so that a fuller discussion can be generated and disagreements explored.
4. The leader helps the group to process its diverse information and perspectives.
5. The leader structures sessions so that a period of idea generation is separated from a period of idea evaluation.
6. The leader structures sessions so as to keep the group focused on its issues and its goals and not lost in conflict or side issues.
7. The leader helps the group focus on its mutual interests rather than emphasizing conflict; the leader helps the group realize

that its mutual interests can be served through the open expression of disagreement as long as the long-range goals are kept clearly in mind.

8. The leader helps those with minority or unpopular opinions to express them; the leader acts in ways to protect dissenters from harrassment, ridicule, or rejection.

A Conclusion.   Although any member can serve leadership functions, the designated leader or organizer bears a special responsibility to help a group use its resources as assets rather than as liabilities. A review of the listed leader behaviors that help a characteristic such as diversity become an asset rather than a liability suggests the importance of the leader's attitude, philosophy, and style. Basically, a person's style of leadership affects whether a particular characteristic of a group will become an asset or a liability. This suggests that it is important to understand the concept of leadership *style*.

LEADERSHIP STYLE

When we talk about a style of leadership, we are simply referring to the typical ways in which a person takes on the leadership role within a group. Leadership style can be seen to be a result of the person's underlying theory of human nature. Leadership style, in turn, results in a particular set of consequences for the group that is being led. We can organize our thinking about leadership style through the following diagram:

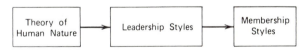

Figure 10-1. Antecedents and outcomes of leadership style.

The diagram indicates that the theory of human nature a person maintains will influence the particular style of group leadership he or she adopts. That style, in turn, will influence the ways in which the members of the group behave together. To more fully appreciate this diagram and its implications, we must begin our inquiry with an examination of some underlying theories of human nature that are related to leadership styles.

Theories of Human Nature

Several years ago, McGregor (1960) introduced the idea that people varied in their conception of human nature. He spoke of Theory X and Theory Y conceptions. The Theory X person, according to McGregor, believes that other people

1. Dislike work and so avoid it if they can
2. Must be coerced, controlled, and even threatened into working
3. Have little ambition or stomach for responsibility and so really enjoy being directed and strongly led.

The Theory Y person believes that

1. Effort expended in work is as natural and pleasurable as effort expended in play
2. People are capable of exercising self-direction and self-control once they feel committed to certain objectives and goals
3. People not only learn to accept but actively seek areas in which they can be autonomous and responsible.

The implication of this theory of leadership practice is fairly self-evident. People subscribing to Theory X would be likely to engage in what Maier (1970) terms a leadership style of "persuasive selling." They would believe it essential to direct and to control others. They would not trust others to be responsible or to be able to take any initiative and would see their own role therefore as demanding a high level of control, dominance, and supervision. Theory Y leaders, by contrast, would be more likely to engage in a "problem-solving" style of leadership. Basically, their goal would focus on helping the group solve problems rather than on accepting the leaders' own pre-formed opinion.

Self-Fulfilling Prophecy. An intriguing quality of these philosophies and their associated styles of group leadership is their self-fulfilling nature. That is, it is not surprising to find that group members led by Theory X leaders require direction and close supervision; they seem to lack initiative and appear unable to do things on their own without the leader's presence and guidance. The leader's theory about human nature is thereby validated by the group's behavior. That this leader's own style of leadership may have contributed to this style of membership often escapes notice. There is good reason to believe, however, that a particular leadership style gives rise to a particular membership style; the latter is usually one that confirms the leader's ideas about human nature and thus a propecy is fulfilled and a leadership style justified.

The Democratic, Autocratic, and Laissez-Faire Leadership Styles

One of the best known descriptions of leadership styles was formulated some years ago by Lewin, Lippitt, and White (see Lippitt & White, 1958). It differentiates between a member-centered problem-solving style termed *democratic*, a leader-centered "persuasive selling" style termed *autocratic*, and a noncentered style termed *laissez-faire*.

Democratic Leadership Style. This member-centered leadership style tends to follow from the Theory Y concept of human nature; it emphasizes the utilization of the resources within groups that are available and must be tapped. Its design is to create a climate within which members can openly express themselves, share their diversity without fear of rejection or excessive conflict, explore their different skills and talents, and build upon these in accomplishing their mutual tasks. Democratic leaders adopt a problem-solving perspective; their goal is to help members achieve their own ends rather than sell the group the leaders' views or ideas.

The democratic style is very active; its mission basically is to facilitate the members' participation in decisions, formulating and evaluating policy, considering alternatives, taking action. The leader's efforts are directed toward including all members in the groups activities and decisions. Some specific aspects of this style include the following:

1. The leader works with the members in developing plans that are agreeable to everyone rather than telling members exactly what they are to do and how they are to do it.

2. The leader's statements are intended to guide rather than to direct.

3. The leader takes on responsibility for helping the group evaluate its progress; also intervenes to help the group keep to its agenda and not stray too far from its goals.

4. The leader gives expert information only when it is pertinent to the situation at hand; he or she does not use expertise irrelevantly to gain status.

5. The leader supports spontaneous shifts in direction and the methods that emerge from within the group that all agree are within the limits defined by the group.

(from Deutsch, Pepitone & Zander, 1948)

An Example. One of the six members of a university school of nursing teaching team was designated "team leader" by the university. The first six months or so of this team's life together was spent primarily in working on intra-team issues of communication and relationships. When the group was first convened, most of the team members sat back and waited to be told what to do. There was great pressure on the leader from the members to adopt an autocratic rather than a democratic leadership style. The university administration, in turn, applied pressure on the team leader to accept certain directives they handed down and to work to get the team to agree to these policy directives. But the team leader strongly believed in the importance of the democratic leadership style. She resisted both the team's and the administration's efforts to convert her to a more autocratic mode of group leadership. She spent much time and effort working with the team democratically, in getting members to accept their responsibility for the team's functioning, in getting members to communicate and share their ideas openly and without fear of rejection or ridicule. The result was the formation of a highly cohesive working unit. The team became highly innovative in its curriculum planning and implementation, and thus gained a positive reputation as one of the most cohesive and productive teams at the school. The extra time invested in developing the team paid off in a high yield for team members, other faculty at the university, and the students in nurse's training.

Autocratic Leadership Style. The autocratic style is leader-centered rather than member-centered. Autocratic leaders feel that they know best; their main task is conceived as convincing others of the correctness of their own views: they engage in "persuasive selling." They stifle disagreement within the group unless it helps them better achieve their own personal ends (a divide-and-conquer strategy). They tend to be secretive in their dealings with members, believing that members should be prevented from knowing too much. Keeping group members in the dark about what the goals are and what the relation is between present activities and these goals is a typical technique of autocratic leaders. Such people are proficient at covering over issues that might thwart achievement of their own ends for the group. The group, for them, is not a locus of human resources that need to be tapped but a means of accomplishing personal goals.

This separation of members' knowledge of activities from group goals is often noted by hospital staff. One group, for example, was asked to provide ideas regarding better ways to keep hospital records updated. A committee was formed to gather these ideas, which were then reviewed at staff meetings, agreed upon, and given to the leader to be forwarded to the central administration. Four weeks later a directive arrived from central administration detailing a new set of policies for record keeping. The new policies had no relation whatsoever to those proposed by the staff that was to implement them. In other words, these staff members were "invited" to participate but were then kept in the dark about what happened to their ideas.

The autocratic style need not be nor typically is a hostile or aggressive style (e.g., Bradford & Lippitt, 1961). Such leaders can be very personable, even warm and friendly. However, their essential message to the members says, "Let me handle it, I know best." Hard-boiled autocrats seek to secure discipline and conformity to their directive without questioning; the more benevolent autocrat appears to be interested in group members and appears to work closely with them (a pat on the back, a friendly smile of reassurance). The autocratic message remains much the same: "You did it my way and I'm pleased." The autocrat tends to foster excessive dependency on his or her way; they are the group's central focus, and without them no action can be taken, no decisions made.

A frequent variant on the autocratic style is found among people who use what appears to be a democratic, member-centered approach but only as a more complex and sophisticated method for covering over their own persuasive purposes. These people may appear to court member opinion and appear to be open to listening, but only in the name of being a better salesperson; their true interests are in reality to convince the group about their views rather than to help the members develop and express and work with their own resources.

Dr. Rimose is the chief of out-patient services; he is an engaging, genuinely delightful medical man, highly respected in his field. In staff meetings, he always invites new ideas; he appears to listen to all complaints that are sent his way. Yet he makes all the decisions and does everything precisely in his own way. The staff members are personally fond of Dr. Rimose, but they know that their ideas have little chance of being seriously considered or implemented by him if they are contrary to the doctor's own wishes. The meetings are very amicable, and decisions are made with little trouble or hesitation; the decisions, of course, are always in support of Dr. Rimose's own policies. On the surface the group appears to be very well-organized, happy, and effective. However, things are not what they seem. One member of the staff, Dr. Cutler, the assistant director feels belittled by Dr. Rimose's leadership style and methods. Dr. Cutler is not sure that she can remain, even though she likes the position and works well. She feels the need for greater sharing of authority. Ms. O'Connor, the head nurse, smiles on the outside but seethes internally. She constantly brings her complaints to the director of nursing. Her complaints, like those of Dr. Cutler, involve having little or no say in the policies that Dr. Rimose determines. The department Dr. Rimose heads generates many ideas (all of them his), but has great difficulty in implementing these ideas. The staff says yes, but becomes passively aggressive, dragging their feet in complying with the decisions. Somehow, the records never quite get done; the new admissions procedure is never quite completed, and so forth.

Laissez-Faire Leadership Style. This third type of leadership style is neither member- nor leader-centered; rather, it is almost a noncentered style. As the French word suggests, its essence is simply to let things alone to develop as they will. Laisse-faire leaders tend to be a bit withdrawn from any active involvement in the group; they take non-directiveness to its extreme. They do not seek to engage members in discussions, or to facilitate member involvement and participation; nor do they take the total burden into their own hands. They sit back and act as though everything will eventually work out. This style is characterized by the tendency simply to let things drift; clear goals for the group are never formulated; decisions are not made; ongoing evaluation of group process is missing.

This is a style that one sees increasingly among those who have come to distrust all forms of authority and who seem to feel that the best type of leader is the nonleader. Unfortunately, the results of such a style tend to be confusion and nonfunctioning. Or members' frustration builds and they turn to an autocratic member of the group to provide them directive leadership.

Ms. Brady, a nursing instructor, was the group leader for fifteen baccalaureate students in their first term. These students began with no idea of nursing process. At her supervisory sessions, Ms. Brady reported that her group was so relaxed and so together that they really did not need any type of leadership or direction from her. She just let them do anything they wanted: "Today, for example, I sat back and read a newspaper while two students studied for a meds exam, three wandered in and out over the two-hour session, and some others talked. It was really great." Her idea of leadership was to let the group do whatever they wanted. The group never became a cohesive unit; they never really talked together about nursing or about much of anything. They learned nothing.

A Summary Diagram. The following diagram (Fig. 10–2) summarizes a continuum of leadership behavior from the extreme of leader-centeredness to the extreme of member-centeredness.

THE RESULTS OF DIFFERENT STYLES: FROM LEADERSHIP STYLE TO MEMBERSHIP STYLE

We have painted a picture of the various styles of leadership in rather broad strokes, leaving aside the many individual variations that are possible. We can also paint an equally general picture of some of the major consequences that derive from each of the styles. These have been alluded to in several examples. What is important to realize is the degree to which a particular leadership style *produces* a corresponding membership style, even one that all parties may agree is not desirable.

Following is a summary of the membership styles that derive from the three major types of leadership behavior.

Democratic Membership Style   *Summary*

1. Members display a high degree of enthusiasm for their work and considerable involvement and commitment to their work and to their group.
2. A high degree and quality of productivity is generated, giving members the added satisfaction of having participated significantly in producing something of high quality.
3. There is a high degree of group cohesiveness, sense of comradeship, and good morale.
4. Members learn to take on personal responsibilities and to take the initiative; they are able to work effectively even when the

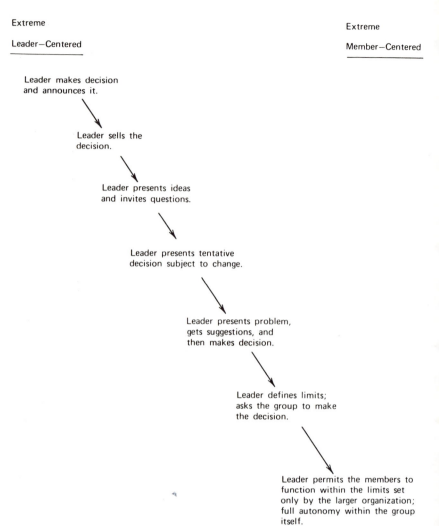

Figure 10-2. Leadership styles (Tannenbaum & Schmidt, 1958).

leader is late or absent. In the original Lippitt and White research, for example, members continued working when the leader had to leave the room; likewise, they began working even when the leader arrived late. This behavior indicated their general independence from the leader and their ability to take on individual responsibility and initiative for themselves.

5. Members begin to learn leadership skills and effective leader behavior.

6. There is a high degree of motivation and participation. There are few, if any, apathetic members.

Autocratic Membership Style

1. There is much resentment and bitterness over having submitted to the leader. There may be incipient revolts which only the presence of the leader can contain. This has been described by Lippitt and White as a pot ready to boil over; only the leader's presence can keep the lid on.
2. No one takes on any personal responsibility or shows an initiative; there is much buck-passing and resistance to the work. Lippitt and White's data indicate, for example, that members of autocratically led groups do not begin work or continue work without the presence of the leader to spur them on.
3. Symptoms of irritability and resentment show up increasingly: lateness, petty anger over minor matters; apathy. Lippitt and White's data indicate how members scapegoat one another or scapegoat an outsider who comes into the room while the leader is absent. The scapegoat is used as the target for the anger members fear to express directly toward the leader.
4. Productivity may be high, but constant surveillance and supervision are required to maintain it. Turnover may be substantial, resulting in long-term reduction of productive efficiency.
5. Members fail to learn how to function independently, thus few new ideas or innovations develop.
6. Group morale and cohesiveness are low.

Laissez-Faire Membership Style

1. There is low member morale and minimal interest in the task or in the group.
2. There is low group cohesiveness and minimal member concern for one another.
3. Work tends to be sloppy and inefficient; productivity is low.
4. Irritability and unrest tend to be general and unfocused, often building around a feeling of confusion and frustration about the group's drift and inability to get off the ground.

5. There may be much scapegoating as members search around for someone or something to blame for their frustrations.

6. Members are not trained in any leadership skills. They tend to withdraw from active involvement; they become apathetic and bored.

SOME OBJECTIONS TO THE DEMOCRATIC STYLE

There are some who object to the democratic, member-centered style. It sounds good in theory, critics say, but has little place in practice. In particular, some feel that medical and nursing practice are founded on a hierarchy of expertise in which member participation can only weaken the expert's proper role and result in poor work. In this section we will examine three related answers to these objections concerning the democratic leadership style. The first examines the need for *flexibility* in leadership style; the second investigates the difficulties involved when one person tries to take on *opposing styles* of leadership; the third looks at the effects of leadership style on the *acceptance* of decisions.

Flexibility

When To Be More Directive. There are settings and circumstances in which a clearly defined line of authority is necessary; in which one decision maker must integrate information, decide, and get others to follow his or her directives. Some research (e.g., Fiedler, 1967) has suggested the importance of a more autocratic leadership style when tasks are highly structured, when the leader has substantial member support and acceptance for his or her ideas, or when the group's situation is such that without strong direction it will fall apart.

For example, on a highly structured task, one in which the alternatives are limited (in the extreme, there may be only one choice to make), a more directive approach may be warranted. Excessive member involvement in the decision process would only serve to delay the inevitable or so confuse members that their cooperation is actually less than it would have been with a more directive leader. However, when the task has many alternatives, when much information is needed, when issues of value and ethics are involved, the more democratic approach is warranted. This would seem to be the case in much work within the health professions: different points of view regarding patient management exist; no single clear solution is present; information from several different sources (e.g., medical, nursing, social workers, etc.) is needed for proper patient care.

The Issue of Rigidity.   The problem, of course, is that most persons who engage in leadership functions tend to rigidly adhere either to one style or the other, thereby disregarding the unique characteristics of the situation and the task. In this case, one may be either rigidly democratic or rigidly autocratic in style, rather than adopting an approach that fits the special circumstances that are involved. Typically, however, it is rigid adherence to a Theory X, autocratic style that dominates even in situations and with tasks for which this is not essential and may even be detrimental. It is less typical to find persons behaving in rigidly democratic ways even on tasks in which only one solution is possible.

The skills that are required for democratic leadership are much more demanding and complex than those required for the other styles. In the case of autocratic leadership, one must have a good sense of his or her own position and then work to persuade others or demand that others adopt it. In the democratic style, however, a person must basically work with group process: i.e., adopt the problem-solving perspective and be oriented toward the utilization of members as resources for group action.

The democratic style demands that leaders be willing to reorient their own ideas so that they are no longer concerned with personally winning, or not losing, a point. In the name of winning, many a leader or member has turned to the autocratic style. If it is important for me to have my ideas recognized as originating with me, if it is important for me to be able to say at the conclusion of the meeting that the group has adopted my platform and done what I suggested, then I am not likely to be able to do more than try to steer the group along the lines I wish for them. But if I can accept neither winning nor losing—that is, if I can agree that the process of member involvement in discussion and decision is more important than my own ideas—then I can begin to act in ways that help members explore, examine, and evaluate their own points of view and suggestions.

Assuming Opposing Leadership Styles

Several years ago, Bales (we previously considered some of his works) suggested that we are not likely to find what he termed a "great-man" leader (see Bales, 1955; 1958; Borgatta, et al., 1954). By this he meant that few people have the capabilities of simultaneously serving what he termed the task functions and the socioemotional functions of the group. Task functions have to do with getting the work done; they may require a leader to be directive or at least to focus on what are at times the less pleasant aspects of accomplishing goals. Socioemotional functions have to do with the human relations side of group work, with emphasis on group harmony and cohesiveness. It was Bales' contention, based both on theory and his research, that only rarely can one and the same person press a group on to do its tasks and simultaneously help group members deal with interpersonal issues.

One way of thinking about this difficulty is to assume that effective work on the group's task usually necessitates some division of labor: individuals take on different aspects of the total job that has to be done. These differences, in turn, highlight the distinctions between the members. A kind of status hierarchy tends to emerge, and with it invidious comparisons, competition, and jealousy. Socioemotional issues, on the other hand, tend to involve ways in which members are similar—things they share in common: e.g., equality of pay, of respect, of status.

Bales suggested that it is very difficult for one person to push members toward inequality on the one hand (by focusing on task issues) and at the same time push them toward equality (by focusing on socioemotional issues). Hence, no "great-person" leader—no one person who can serve both sets of functions for the group. As we have already noted, the autocratic style may indeed get members to work on their tasks; yet in its failure to deal with interpersonal issues, this method may create tensions and resentments that in the long run thwart group effectiveness. But what about a more democratic style?

Feedback Ratio.   As part of one of his investigations, Bales (1958) developed the concept of the *feedback ratio.* This was conceived as a measure of the degree to which a person who sends out considerable communication to others (e.g., talks a great deal and seems to dominate) allows communication back from others. A high feedback ratio indicates that there is a reasonable proportionality between what is sent out and what is allowed back in return. A low ratio, by contrast, indicates that someone sends out much, but allows little back. Bales posited that persons with a high feedback ratio were more likely to be "great-person" leaders than those with low ratios. In other words, the leader who courts considerable participation from members is more likely to satisfy both task and socioemotional demands. This, of course, is descriptive of the democratic, member-centered leadership style.

The leader with a low feedback ratio does not approximate the "great-person" leader; he or she tends to dominate a discussion, contributing much to task issues while failing to consider socioemotional functions. In that both sets of functions must be dealt with for a group to work together effectively in the long run, leaders with a low feedback ratio are not helpful. In fact, they contribute to socioemotional conflicts by their domination. This, of course, is one of the outcomes of the more autocratic style.

The Issue of Acceptance

Maier (1970) points out what initially appears to be a paradox, one that seems especially at issue in the health professions. Leaders often feel that they hold the key to high-quality solutions to the problems and issues within the groups they lead. They sense that they really do know what is best by virtue of their training, experience, and expertise. As they may experience it, the only problem is how to get others to accept their expertise. The paradox arises when the issue of acceptance is analyzed. Here it is important to note first that more decisions are ineffective because they lack the acceptance of those who must adopt and implement them than because they lack quality. Second, acceptance may best be gained if the efforts to sell one's expertise to others is abandoned and those others are brought into more equal partnership: i.e., via a democratic leadership style.

The issue of leadership cannot be divorced from the issue of acceptance. It does us little good to hold all the expertise and wisdom in the world if others do not accept the fruits of this wisdom. Health professionals may fervently believe in their own correctness and expertise and be unable to understand why their patients may fail to heed their advice except when under direct surveillance: e.g., they take their medications when we watch them, but not on their own.

ACCEPTANCE AND THE PSYCHOLOGY
OF LEADERSHIP

The issue of acceptance brings us directly up against the psychological side of leadership. Several ideas proposed by Kelman (1958; 1961) are particularly helpful at this point; they focus our attention on three processes involved in the acceptance or nonacceptance of leadership: compliance, identification, and internalization.

Compliance

Compliance refers to acceptance of leadership based primarily on either fear of the consequences for not accepting (e.g., punishment) or the promises of rewards for accepting. In the case of compliance, the group member's acceptance or rejection hinges on the leader's being around to observe that person's behavior. To promise the patient a reward if she follows our advice to cough, however painful it may be, means that we must witness her coughing so that we can reward her appropriately for her compliance. Punishment works in much the same way. Compliance under the threat of punishment for noncompliance requires surveillance. This mode of gaining acceptance is very inefficient; it demands that the leader remain around to observe members' behaviors. Surely leaders have better things to do with their time.

Compliance tends to be the essential psychological process involved in the autocratic leadership style. As long as the leader is around to observe and supervise directly, the work gets done. But acceptance as compliance demands constant leader presence, supervision, and surveillance. Leaving aside all matters of resentment and anger, acceptance based on compliance requires members' constant dependence on the leader and discourages the development of autonomous ways of thinking and behaving.

Identification

This second process involves an acceptance of leadership based on the member's attraction to the leader or their wanting to be like the leader; i.e., the leader represents a person with whom they identify and so his or her leadership is accepted in order to maintain that relationship. Although identification may appear to require the same high degree of surveillance as compliance, what typically occurs is an acceptance of the influence without the leader's immediate presence. The leader is carried around within members' heads as one who figuratively says, "If I knew what you were doing now, how would I feel?" Identification may also provoke negative acceptance if the identification itself is negative; that is, if a member's identification is with the opposite of the leader's own characteristics. In this case, rejection rather than acceptance is likely.

Acceptance based on identification is possible if the autocratic leader is benevolent and caring even though domineering; it is also likely to occur with a well-liked leader, someone whom members try to please.

Groupthink. Irving Janis (1973; also see Chapter 4 of this text) used the term *groupthink* to describe a process within many kinds of decision-making groups in which loyalty toward a group leader combines with members' desires to reach consensus at any cost, to produce a highly cohesive but typically uncritical problem-solving group. A leader who builds acceptance on identification is very likely to find groupthink as the result. In such groups, members fail to critically examine each other's suggestions; nor are the leader's ideas open to much scrutiny. Rather, all criticism is avoided and a cozy, friendly atmosphere is sought. Decisions reached within such a group are likely not to have been put to the test of careful member evaluation.

In Janis' view, the antidote to this tendency for groups with high leader loyalty (i.e., identification) to engage in groupthink consists of several elements. First, there is a need to break the group's isolation from other groups with other points of view—perhaps by testing all group decisions out in a larger context with nongroup members before putting them into action. Second, the leader must play an instrumental role in helping override the demanding pressures that stem from members' loyalty and identification. Thus, leaders of a highly cohesive group have a special obligation to enact the role in a democratic manner; to withhold stating their own position until members' positions have been introduced; to help bring alternatives and unpopular possibilities to light; to become a devil's advocate for the group's decisions.

The concept of groupthink reminds us that groups that are cohesive, amiable, that hang together and seem to act as a single unit loyal to an appointed, formal leader, may not be effective in the sense of accomplishing high-quality solutions to the problems and issues with which they deal. Quality derives from the critical examination of alternatives; this demands that alternatives be prosposed, examined, and tested for their consequences before final policy is established and implemented. Disagreement is therefore essential and cannot be seen by the leader or other members as a symptom of disloyalty. It is this tendency to view disagreement as a sign of personal rejection or disloyalty to the "team" or the leader that thwarts effective, quality group work and leads to groupthink.

Internalization

This process involves a form of acceptance in which the recommendations of the leader fit the members' own systems of belief and knowledge. Internalization tends to require minimal surveillance; once members have heard the arguments and evaluate them against their own standards, they come to accept the ideas because of their fit or congruence with what they think is true, right, and proper. Or, of course, if the recommendations do not fit, they are rejected.

Psychologically speaking, therefore, acceptance involves three separate processes, each of which has rather different implications for leadership. Acceptance as compliance requires leaders to emphasize their power to reward or to punish and to observe whether or not persons have complied. This builds upon unilateral control; leaders hope to coerce others into complying with their suggestions.

With identification, the leader hopes to capitalize on members' attraction for him or her. The leader becomes a model for members' behavior; they accept the leader's ideas in order to affirm their identifications.

Leaders who build upon their credibility and expertise, who emphasize the reasonableness of their ideas and the relevance of the values expressed by these ideas, are attempting to gain acceptance by means of internalization. This process is more compatible than either of the other two with a democratic style of leadership. Such leaders do not seek to make capital on their power to punish or reward nor on members' idealizations of their personality; rather, they seek to persuade, as any other member might, by the relevance of their ideas to members' own systems of belief and knowledge. Insofar as their recommendations and ideas fail to fit members' own beliefs, they will not be accepted; and we add, perhaps they should not be.

In other words, leaders who are willing to fail, to have members reject what they think is true because the members' own conceptions conflict with the leader's, are behaving in a more truly democratic style. Indeed, such people try to persuade members, but do not call upon compliance or identification to gain acceptance; democratic leaders are open to having their own judgments altered in and through personal interaction with members. The influence process is much more bilateral.

As we have noted in this discussion of acceptance, the issue is not an idle one of purely theoretical interest. No group can function meaningfully nor for long as an effective group without member acceptance of the process and procedures that are used. A leader basically fails to lead if he or she must gain acceptance entirely on the basis of either compliance or identification. With the former, leadership is built upon force and can only prove to be unstable in the long run and highly dissatisfying for members. With the latter, leadership is built upon the unswerving loyalty and allegiance of followers; and few have the great wisdom, unswerving patience, or foresight to serve well those who have become so dependent on them. The excesses of such loyalty, of course, also thwart carefully considered, critical group evaluation; the process that tends to result is *groupthink*.

LEADERSHIP: TRANSFERENCE AND COUNTERTRANSFERENCE

In Chapter 5, we noted the importance that psychoanalytic theory attached to the unconscious relationships that formed between a group's members and its leader. These unconscious bonds of attachment involving the members' feelings about the leader are referred to as *transference*; when they involve the leader's feelings about the members, they are referred to as *countertransference*. Basically, any person, whether he or she is the formal leader or a member who performs significant leadership functions can become the target of transference and in turn experience qualities of countertransference.

A Potent Label

As we will see, transference relationships tend to be very strong and difficult to overcome. These kinds of distortions in relationship tend to occur between members and anyone who is given the role of group leader. Often, just the mere label or designation group leader" is sufficient to bring out some of these unconscious connections between members and that person. If individuals given the title of leader are not aware of the concept of transference, they may suddenly find themselves the recipient of many unusual feelings and expectations which they are neither able to understand nor appreciate. Often, they become confused and puzzled by members' expectations for them and their behavior. They cannot fathom, for example, why it is that whatever they do may please some and infuriate others. Such leaders find it difficult to grasp why their words, often uttered casually and without much thought, seem to carry a heavy burden of weight and meaning. They may soon become fearful of talking, lest they say something wrong or that offends a member. They sense a degree of responsibility that they are not sure they deserve or want. In other words, the potency of transference often escapes the prospective group leader who doesn't realize that even the label "leader" carries with it a role and triggers various unconscious processes in others.

The Meaning of Transference

When we speak of transference, we are describing members' unconscious tendencies to relate to the leader in terms of some qualities that they require persons in authority to possess; these are usually not the qualities that the leader actually possesses. In this sense, therefore, members transfer onto the leader their projections regarding persons in authority. As we already noted, groupthink derives in part from a shared transference in which members become blindly obedient to those in authority and accept their ideas without critical evaluation. Transference within groups, however, encompasses blind rejection as well as blind acceptance.

Leaders may notice that some members use whatever the leader proposes as a springboard for their own needs to reject authority. Such persons do not critically examine the leader's proposals, but appear to reject them instinctively, reflexively, and out of hand. This kind of automatic rejection, similar to automatic acceptance, can mean that a transference relationship has evolved. It should be apparent that effective group functioning and quality work derive from the use of more rational and critical human capacities; thus, the interposition of transference between members and their leader thwarts group effectiveness.

Member Types and Transference

Several years ago, Bennis and Shepard (1956) proposed an analysis of members in terms of their tendencies to transfer excessive dependency or excessive counterdependency onto leaders and other persons in positions of authority. *Dependent* people relate to authorities in a passive and submissive manner. As group members, they need strong and directive leadership; they feel most comfortable when the leader enacts a more autocratic than democratic style. It is not unusual for many leaders to be attracted to these kinds of members; their obedience and apparent uncritical acceptance of the leader's proposals can prove pleasing to anyone hoping for consensus around his or her own ideas. But in their uncritical dependency on those in authority, such dependent people serve less to facilitate a group than to inhibit its effectiveness. The "yes-saying" member may give the leader momentary peace of mind, but fails to provide the kind of critical sensitivity that is required for quality work to emerge.

Counterdependent people compulsively reject whatever organization, structure, initiative, or suggestions are proposed by the leader. Such group members view authorities with suspicion as dangerous, as threats to their full freedom and autonomy; they act uncritically to reject proposals. Their mode does not provide alternatives but rather knocks down whatever is being proposed. In this way, therefore, they hardly can be said to be helpful resources. Often group leaders, recognizing the counterdependents' tendencies, play up to them and try to curry their favor; this wastes much time and energy in placating members whose unconscious needs require a constant rejection of all authority.

Handling Transferences

These are extreme descriptions; it is not likely that any single person will be entirely dependent or entirely counterdependent. And it is difficult to say just which pattern makes the leadership role more difficult.

If our discussion pertained to a therapy group, our advice would urge the leader to help members work through their transferences as a key ingredient to their move toward good health. However, we are not dealing with therapy groups. Working through members' unconscious transferences toward the leader can be inappropriate in many settings. The leader's task, therefore, involves spotting members who appear to be caught by their own transferences (i.e., trapped into a compulsive dependent or counterdependent mode of interacting with the authority) and members whom Bennis and Shepard term *independents*: i.e., persons who seem not so compulsive in their transferences, who seem better able to respond appropriately rather than projecting their own unconscious needs so blatantly onto the leader.

Independents provide a continuing check for the leader on his or her own ideas and proposals; they provide a resource for others to model. Although members who are in conflict over authority may not gain much insight into the basis of this conflict, they can learn the ways in which effective member functioning can occur by observing how the independents deal with leadership. In this way, they can reduce their own transference on the leader and begin to play a more effective role within the group. The leader can be instrumental in this endeavor by building his or her approach around those members who appear to have less conflict and who are less apt to transfer their unconscious dependencies or counterdependencies.

Reality Testing. Yalom (1975), while dealing primarily with therapy groups, nevertheless offers another useful way for leaders to minimize the negative effects of transference. Basically, in that transferences involve distorted perceptions of leaders' behavior, a leader can act to bring a clear touch of reality to member's perceptions. Leaders who in truly autocratic fashion act as though they were indeed omnipotent can readily feed members distorted perceptions of authority. The dependents will see such leaders as infallible, as their true savior; the counterdependents will have their worst fantasies realized as they encounter someone who actively seeks to control them and prevent them from being autonomous.

To counter this tendency, a good leader would have to help restore members' more accurate perceptions by appearing frankly as the more fallible and less omniscient human being that he or she actually is. In other words, a leader can either foster transference or thwart it. Transference builds upon distortions of the reality of authority; it can be remedied by a confrontation with the reality of the leader.

Leaders who can confess ignorance and confusion when indeed they are ignorant or confused, for example, help bring members' perceptions back to reality. To say, "I don't know" when one really doesn't know, rather than formulating an answer just to appear good and on top of things, can likewise help shatter members' fantasies based on needs involving transference.

A leader who seriously tries to enlist the involvement of members in the group, who is genuinely affected by members even while affecting them (i.e., a more equal exchange rather than a unilateral control), will likewise help shatter distorted views of the leader as all-knowing and all-powerful. Members will come to see the leader who accepts their influence in realistic terms.

Countertransference

While members form unconscious attitudes toward the leader, leaders also are prone to countertransference; that is, they can project onto members some of their own conflicts and unconscious needs. Some leaders require groups that will permit them to lead in a directive and autocratic manner; only in this way can their own needs for power be met. Any hint of disapproval or disagreement is met with quick response on their part; they experience disagreements as threats to their power.

Much the same can be said about leaders who demand approval; they may be insecure in their role and gauge their effectiveness in terms of how much love, attention, and approval they receive from their group members. In order to gain this approval rather than to accomplish effectiveness as a group, such leaders play upon members' feelings; they overemphasize socioemotional factors to the detriment of task issues. Such leaders would rather be liked than have an effective (e.g., critically thinking and acting) group. They adopt a leadership style that encourages others to adore them, to need and depend on them, in the extreme, even to worship them. In doing this, they fail to carry out their leadership functions.

Dealing with Countertransference

It is especially difficult to deal with countertransferences. Members can and do act in ways that feed leaders' own needs for approval, love, and power. It is often difficult for the leader to see clearly what is actually taking place. When members agree with our proposals it is easy to find ourselves drawn to them. They may praise our ways of organizing the group and leading it, drawing us even closer toward them. We soon forget that our functions are best served when we can bring together a diverse range of members' opinions, when we can facilitate having these opinions carefully analyzed and critically tested. It is difficult not to be seduced by our patients or group members into believing their fantasies about us, especially if they come to transfer great power upon us as their healer and leader. We are flattered; we desperately want to believe them to be correct.

All leaders are subject to countertransference; just as all members are prone to transference. There are no quick and easy remedies;

awareness and sensitivity to the several possibilities we have discussed is a vital first step, however. The more fully aware leaders are of themselves and their purposes, of the pleasures and the displeasures of leading, the better they can be in spotting those moments when the grip of countertransference begins to tighten and stifle their effectiveness as group leaders.

SUMMARY AND CONCLUSIONS

This chapter has reviewed and examined some of the major issues, styles, and effects of group leadership. The discussion was opened with the proposition that leadership is best understood in terms of functions that are performed rather than in terms of a specific person or set of personality traits. We noted, however, that a specific person may be designated leader and will have many of these functions to perform; but members also can and do perform leadership functions and usually should be encouraged to do so.

We next considered some of the assets and the liabilities that can occur within groups and related these to the particular style of leadership that is employed. Particular styles can make what would otherwise be an asset a liability and vice versa. Leadership styles derive from the individual's philosophy of human nature and result in particular kinds of membership responses, or membership styles. We considered two philosophies, Theory X (a more autocratic and controlling perspective) and Theory Y (a more humanistic perspective). We examined three leadership styles—democratic, autocratic, and laissez-faire—and the resulting three membership styles. Overall, our evaluation emphasized the benefits that appear to accrue to a more democratic leadership style.

It was noted that there may be several objections to the adoption of a democratic leadership style, especially in the more hierarchical systems in which most health professionals are trained and in which they typically work. We examined objections involving issues of flexibility in style; opposing characteristics that made the adoption of two styles difficult unless one tended to use more democratic means; acceptance of leadership and the various psychological bases of such acceptance. In general, a democratic style, all things considered, has much more merit than alternative styles of group leadership.

The chapter ended with an examination of the complex issues of transference and countertransference that are involved in group leadership. The prospective leader needs to be sensitive to members' transferences, which may make the leadership role puzzling, confusing, and even frightening. We examined ways with which these transferences can be dealt. Finally, the issues of countertransference were discussed, noting the temptations for the leader to believe members' fantasies and to lead in ways that satisfy his or her own needs, often to the detriment of the group's effectiveness. A greater sensitivity to these possibilities and a greater self-awareness is necessary for the good leader. Supervision while training to lead groups will prove to be a helpful antidote to the problems of both transference and countertransference.

11

Techniques of Group Leadership: Processing and Feedback

A review of the functions of leadership suggests the following to be important elements:

- Obtaining and receiving information
- Helping in the diagnosis of group goals, obstacles, and consequences of decision choices
- Facilitating communication
- Helping integrate the various perspectives and alternative possibilities for policy or action that emerge within the group
- Testing and evaluating proposals and decisions

Although these are separable aspects of leadership, more significantly, they all require skills in what we will term *processing.*

THE PROCESSING FUNCTIONS OF LEADERSHIP

Processing requires rather complex perceptual and cognitive abilities in addition to the interpersonal skills it also demands from the group's leader. When we process interactions we focus on the immediate situation that is present here and now. This requires an ability to be at some distance from the immediate, ongoing situation even while actively participating in it. Distance provides the perspective on the immediate present that is necessary for any modification or constructive direction. To process interaction involves being able to reflect upon and evaluate just-completed actions. A diagram of this reflective characteristic of processing appears in Figure 11–1. As the diagram indicates, to process interaction means to pause and make a reflective "loopback" regarding what has just occurred (#1). The processing function of leadership means that people must be able to engage in this continuous reflective appraisal.

For example, suppose we are dealing with a group of nurses who are learning a new technique as part of their in-service training program. As we participate with the group in learning this technique, we also attend to the ongoing interaction that exists within the group. We may observe, for example, that some of the nurses recently out of school are already familiar with the technique, while several who received their training many years earlier are not familiar with it. We may also note that these older nurses, who occupy a higher-status position within the hospital staff, resent being put into a learning situation in which they are at a disadvantage relative to their more knowledgeable, younger colleagues. This resentment is expressed in many subtle ways: e.g., low attention on their part to the instruction; frequent and somewhat inappropriate joking; negativistic comments toward the whole procedure; tendency to avoid interacting with the younger nursing staff; resistance to being paired with younger staff in learning exercises. Processing, in this case, involves reflecting back on the interaction that is emerging while the teaching session itself occurs.

The interpersonal skills that also comprise the processing function require the leader to intervene appropriately in giving the group feedback based on this reflective evaluation. That is, the leader must continuously monitor the group in here-and-now terms. The information obtained from monitoring (#2) must be fed back to the group so that it can become a useful resource in the group's ongoing deliberations and interaction (#3). Interpersonal skills are demanded at this point. Having noted some critical aspect of the group's functioning, in what ways can the leader feed this information back to the group so that it be-

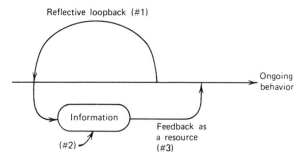

Figure 11-1. Processing the here and now.

comes a resource for the group, something it can use to facilitate or transform its continuing behavior?

The issue facing the group leader in our example is how to provide the group her perceptions regarding their mode of interacting together as a group. Should she simply interrupt the class and inform everyone about what she has seen? Or should she keep quiet and assume that learning will somehow occur regardless of how the group members seem to be relating to one another and to the new technique to be mastered? Should the leader confront one of the senior nurses who seems to be the most resistant, saying something like, "You seem to be openly negativistic about this whole procedure; do you have any sense of why this might be?"

To the extent that the ongoing behavior of the group thwarts accomplishment of its goals (in the example, by frustrating the learning of the new technique), the processing function of leadership requires: (a) perception of this ongoing pattern of group interaction, (b) evaluation of its role in helping or hindering the group, and (c) feedback of this appraisal so that it may be a resource the group can use to correct itself and thereby better accomplish the goals. We will shortly examine both these cognitive and interpersonal aspects of the processing function of leadership in greater detail.

SINGLE-LOOP VS. DOUBLE-LOOP LEARNING

Argyris (1975; 1976; Argyris & Schon, 1974) contrasts what he terms single-loop with double-loop behavior; the skills of double loop-learning are those that involve what we have termed the processing functions of leadership. The example that Argyris chooses to illustrate single-loop behavior is the thermostat, which adjusts the temperature in a room to match a pre-set figure: e.g., 72 degrees. The thermostat receives information from the room, checks that information against the present figure, and feeds the information back so as to turn the heat on or off. In this manner it serves the function of keeping the room at its temperature goal, correcting deviations as necessary. It may appear that this single-loop function is the critical key to good leadership. But Argyris suggests that double-loop behavior is even more important. In this latter case, the thermostat not only evaluates the degree to which the room temperature is on or off its designated target, but goes one step further; it evaluates the target itself. That is, a double-loop thermostat (if one were to exist) would also continuously evaluate whether a room temperature of 68°, 72°, or whatever were a reasonable goal.

Let us not get stuck in describing thermostats. Double-loop behavior within a group requires that the entire context within which the group functions be taken into consideration: that is, evaluation must be continuously made and fed back regarding the variety of alternative goals toward which the group might be heading, the variety of means whereby such goals can be achieved, the variety of consequences that follow from each alternative, the relation between each goal and the members' values, ethics, and responsibilities, and so forth.

Single-loop leader behavior within a group is concerned primarily with how well the group is moving toward a designated goal. This is relevant in many contexts, for example, when there is but one goal and no alternatives to be considered. However, in the usual circumstance, single-loop behavior will only inform the group regarding its deviation from one set goal. A double-loop perspective is needed for the introduction of multiple goals, alternatives, evaluations, and so forth.

Processing thereby involves being able to see where a group is heading, what alternatives are available, what their consequences are, how they may best be achieved, what members feel about these possibilities. All of this must be done while the group is engaged in its activities together; it must all be fed back to the group in order to become a further resource for members' consideration. This is a critical point.

To summarize, we are saying that an important leadership function and skill involves being able to help the group process itself *as it is behaving.* This involves providing a continuous flow of feedback to the group regarding its present situation and the multiplicity of futures toward which it can head. This continuous flow of feedback becomes an additional resource for the group. Knowledge about where it is, where it is going, and where it might be going becomes further material that a group can use in moving most effectively to achieve those ends that it deems essential. And one of the most important functions of leadership involves facilitating this ongoing processing of group behavior.

THE PERCEPTUAL AND INTERPERSONAL
SKILLS OF PROCESSING

LEADER: Let's stop for a few minutes now and take a look at our meeting today. We will want to see if we can describe what has gone on here, to analyze what we have done and how we feel about it. We may also want to take some time to make suggestions for changes that we would like to see.

MEMBER J: I noted that you (pointing to the leader) tried on several occasions to get us to summarize the points we had been making; but for the most part we seemed to ignore that and just continue with the particular point we wanted to make.

MEMBER L: I think that we aren't yet ready to summarize; we first need to develop more points and explore them.

MEMBER K: Yes. There are a lot of details and a lot of points still to be made; but I think we should pause now and try to summarize where we have been. I know that it helps me to know what ground I've covered before trying to move ahead.

MEMBER N: You know, I was so involved in what we were talking about that I just didn't think to stop and check on where we were and where we wanted to go.

LEADER: You see, I wasn't certain how to help in this. I felt a bit confused, with so many ideas and suggestions being made. I felt that we needed to stop and try to take stock before going on. Do you have any suggestions you can make to ensure that we build in this feedback and evaluation rather than just going on and not reflecting on our process?

This leader is attempting to help the group process its previous interaction before it continues. In this case, the leader's feedback to the group is the suggestion that members stop and review before moving ahead. The skills required of this leader include both perceptual and interpersonal abilities.

Perceptual Skills and Processing

Before leaders can intervene in the group and help members evaluate their present situations and their future possibilities, they must be able to *perceive* the unfolding ongoing situation. This requires that leaders be able to view themselves and the group with some perspective. As a full participant within the middle of interaction it becomes difficult to see just what is going on. The leader must adopt a somewhat more distant and analytic role, typically referred to as that of *participant-observer*. The leader both participates in the group and at the same time observes his or her own and others' participation. We can represent this in the following diagram (Fig. 11–2).

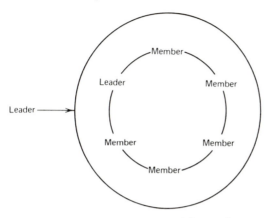

Figure 11-2. Perceiving as a participant-observer.

Dual Roles and Interests.   The diagram illustrates the dual roles and perceptual interests of group leaders who serve the processing function: they are simultaneously within the group as a member and outside the group as an observer viewing themselves and the entire group. One must be inside the group in order to fully understand and appreciate what is being said and experienced by group members; yet one must also be outside the group looking in to see the interaction with some detachment and perspective.

The observer is attentive to patterns of interaction that can be visible only with distance and perspective: e.g., noting that whenever Mary speaks to George, she acts in a deferential manner; or that Sally seems to insist on calling attention to herself, thereby drawing the group away from its other activities in order to attend to Sally. Observers are attentive to the here and now situation. They must actively attempt to see, to experience, and to think in terms of what is taking place here and now. And they must remember that they are part of that here-and-now process.

For example, the leader observes that one member of the group is being negativistic; his actions keep the group fighting and disagreeing. Other members appear restless; one or two express a minor degree of irritation. While noting this behavior, the leader also begins to feel anger arising within herself; the anger is directed toward the negativistic member. Thus, the leader notes something about herself and something about her group: she occupies two roles with two perceptual interests at the same time. It is precisely at this point that the leader requires knowledge of the group process. She must be sensitive to group structures and processes, to theories of group formation and development, to verbal and nonverbal modes of communication. The good observer is a theoretically informed observer.

People generally have difficulty with the idea that they are both participant and observer, occupying dual roles with dual perceptual interests at the same time. The temptation for many persons who work with groups is to adopt one role with only one perceptual interest. Thus, for example, some elect to be all participant and abandon their observer status; others elect to be all observer and abandon their participant status. The former lose a chance to facilitate the group process; they become so caught up in the interaction that they are unable to have the distance necessary to see what is taking place. The latter lose a chance to use their own feelings and experiences as a basis for a better, often more profound understanding of what is taking place in the group. In the example, the leader's awareness of her own anger was a helpful piece of information about the impact of the negativistic member's behavior on herself and on others in the group.

Interpersonal Skills and Processing: Feedback

The leader may be a keen observer; he may be informed and knowledgeable about group process. Yet if his observations and knowledge are to be anything more than of private or abstract theoretical concern, he must be able to translate this information into a resource that the group as a whole can use. The leader in the dialogue at the beginning of this section not only has made observations and analyses of the group, but has also sought to intervene by feeding this material back into the group. They were asked to stop and to review before continuing; in addition, they were asked to develop some procedure for making a review a regular part of their group. In other words, the leader sought to help the group answer several kinds of questions:

1. Where have we been in our discussion thus far?
2. Where do we want to take our discussion?
3. How can we work to ensure that we will ask and answer these questions throughout our future discussions?

In providing this feedback to the group, this leader did not seek to direct the group as such; she sought to provide members with information regarding their whereabouts based on her explicit observations and concerns. This leader, using the democratic style, feels that providing feedback to the group will be sufficient to help members improve themselves and their geoup. That is, she sees her role as being primarily to introduce questions that cause members to focus on their own process of interaction; the assumption is that they can then take this material and use it effectively.

Hypothesis Testing. Another quality of this leader's feedback should be noted. She offers her suggestions in the form of questions and hypotheses that she is testing for their validity. She does not make the assumption that she has the correct appraisal but only that this is her assessment of the group's status. She asks to have her view validated against the views of the others. Her feedback is of the double-loop variety; it is bilateral rather than unilateral as with single-loop behavior. This leader does not *steer* the group, but provides it with ideas to be tested, challenged, and critically evaluated. For example, it is her impression that they should stop and evaluate where they have been; others may disagree. It is her suggestion that they try to build in some procedure for ongoing evaluation; others may disagree.

It may appear that pausing to process a group's behavior takes valuable time away from the important business at hand. Time, to be sure, is not a luxury that we can spend freely. Some groups do not have the time to pause and reflect before acting. In the long run, however, quality solutions to difficult problems and acceptance of decisions hinge on the ability of a group to delay its headlong rush toward a goal before it has processed its movement toward that goal. It may appear impractical to pause. But there is hardly anything as impractical as rushing to a judgment that no one can accept, no one can really agree with, no one really wants to implement, and most importantly, from which no one learns enough to become more proficient in group work the next time around.

INTERPERSONAL SKILLS AND PROCESSING: SOME BASIC TECHNIQUES

The main characteristic of processing is to provide feedback to individuals or to the group about behavior and its effects. It is assumed that this feedback can become a resource which the individual or group can use to help evaluate its ongoing actions and make whatever adjustments are felt to be necessary in order to function more effectively.

This is an important assumption. We assume that if people could be more aware of their actions and the consequences of these actions, they could use this information to work more effectively. This assumption is reasonable in most cases; there is no guarantee, however, that sheer awareness will always be effective in producing needed change. Yet without awareness and knowledge of behavior and its effects, there is little chance to adjust and improve individual or group performance.

An Example of the Feedback Process

Feedback, the crux of processing, can be directed toward an individual member as well as to the group as a whole. For example, the leader may notice that whenever Harry speaks in the group, he lowers his voice, averts his gaze downward, shifts his chair, and leans away from others. The leader may also notice that Harry's ideas, though often sound and helpful for the group to consider, are rarely listened to and never openly discussed. It is as though Harry were not present even though he participates frequently. The leader may feed these perceptions back both to Harry and to the group: "I've noticed, Harry, that whenever you speak you look downward, your voice gets very soft and difficult to hear, and you lean away from the rest of us. This gives me the impression that you lack confidence in your suggestions or are fearful about having others respond to them. I notice myself therefore tending to ignore or at least not pay much attention to what, on reflection, I think are some good ideas. I've also noticed that others in group respond to you in this same way. That is, your ideas are not examined or discussed. It is difficult for a group to work with someone's ideas when the person proposing them seems to be so fearful that to challenge or to examine them closely would be a frightening thing. I wonder if others feel this way and if there is something that we can do about this?"

In this example, the leader provides feedback to Harry and to the group. The feedback follows a useful model for both leaders and other members to learn; the model involves asking and providing answers to four key questions:

1. What do I see?
   The feedback concretely describes a behavior or pattern of behavior that has been observed: e.g., looking downward, soft voice, leaning away.
2. How does it affect me?
   The feedback describes the effect of this behavior on the leader

and its possible effect on the group as a whole: e.g., we tend to ignore what are probably some good ideas.

3. Is this perception and its effects shared by others?

   The feedback presents the leader's observations as hypotheses that need to be checked against the perceptions of others: e.g., do others feel this way?

4. What can we do about it?

   The feedback opens the door to using the information as a resource for continued work and problem-solving: e.g., given these observations, what can we all do to change the undesirable situation?

In the example, the leader's impressions were shared by several other group members; they indicated that often they had wanted to respond to Harry but felt his shyness put them off; they were fearful that if they questioned him closely about his suggestions he would be unable to handle things. Harry, in turn, became aware of his behavior and was able to reassure the group that he was strong enough to take criticism—in fact, that he was eager to have the group work with some of his ideas. Both he and the group were able to alter their behavior sufficiently to begin to use Harry's ideas in the group. To be sure, his manner did not suddenly change; he did not become a bold speaker. Rather, he became aware of the manner by which he presented his ideas; he was able to monitor his own behavior and thus could make adjustments accordingly. The group members, in turn, made special efforts to listen to Harry and to critically discuss his ideas. He did not crack under this new challenge, but rather grew more confident about himself and his contributions.

Processing involves giving feedback to individuals or to the group using the four key elements we noted. But what are the various techniques that are available for giving this feedback? We outline and briefly examine several major techniques. In each case, the goal of the technique remains much the same: to provide information about ongoing behavior and its effects so that this information can become a resource for persons to evaluate and use to modify their actions to better accomplish their goals and interests.

Support

Support involves giving the kind of feedback that helps a person or group continue with its ongoing actions by providing a climate of supportive opinion for this continuation. A supportive intervention for the entire group, for example, may be something as simple as the leader's statement: "I think that we are really doing well now; we seem to be working very effectively, generating some excellent proposals and critically examining each."

Unfortunately, we often mistakenly believe that the only proper kind of feedback involves being critical and informing people when they are off target; with support, however, we recognize that much learning can come from being informed about those times when we are on target. The leader can support an individual member by using positive comments to reinforce useful or helpful behaviors: e.g., "Mary's suggestion that we reconsider our early proposal seems to me to be a good idea. I'm not sure that we'll act any differently on it now than we originally did, but it makes good sense for us to stop and re-evaluate some of our earlier ideas in light of where we now are. That was a good idea, Mary."

Supportive comments serve several functions:

1. They inform persons about behaviors that at least the leader feels are on target and helpful; in this way they permit members to learn when they are doing well.

2. They create a climate of greater confidence for expressing unpopular ideas. None of us really wishes to stand forth with suggestions that others will ridicule or reject offhand. A supportive comment can facilitate the expression of unpopular ideas that may indeed gain in popularity once they are expressed. This is a critical function of leadership: to provide a climate within which divergent points of view can be expressed. Much of this climate is produced in and through the use of supportive comments: e.g., "I know that your idea is not popular with this group, but I, for one, am really pleased that you made it. It think it is a kind of thing that we need more of. I'm not sure yet how I feel about your suggestion, but I do know I'm glad you made it and that we can now all consider it."

3. They help the silent or the more fearful members feel that if they speak in the group there will be someone who will recognize and respond to them. Thus, by being supportive, the leader can facilitate greater member participation.

Confrontation

This is a nasty word, one that brings quickly to mind aggressive battles and warfare. Nothing is farther from the truth about confrontation, however. When we confront someone in the group, we do not intend to do battle or wage war; our goal is not aggressive; we do not wish to conquer. Our goal is, as with all forms of proper feedback, to be helpful in presenting behavior and its effects to the individual or the group. Confrontation is a challenge, however; it tends to startle individuals by forcing them to realize something about themselves and their behavior that they might not otherwise have noted or wanted to note. When we confront people, we place them in a sense in front of a mirror—our perceptions of them—and insist that they look into that mirror and see what they might not otherwise wish to see. We can confront an individual or the group as a whole.

For example, the leader may have noted that one member, Jane, seems insistent in taking the group away from its task and onto off-target discussions. Whenever the discussion seems to get going, Jane is sure to be on hand with something else that she would like everyone to talk about. And, given the difficulties in getting started and remaining on target, everyone else seems to delight in conspiring with Jane to discuss matters that avoid their important but difficult tasks at hand. The leader directly confronts Jane with her behavior: "Jane, I think it is important for you and for the rest of us to stop for a moment and consider what you are doing. It is my impression that whenever we get going in our discussion, for some reason you take us on a side trip. You seem unable or unwilling to let us remain on target or to help us remain on target. I think this is something we should stop and deal with." Here the leader directly confronts Jane with her behavior and invites her and the group to consider it further.

Groups and individuals often get themselves trapped into a pattern of interaction that is undesirable but which they refuse or are unable to see and thus cannot deal with. They cannot get themselves out of this trap because they fail even to see that they are in one in the first place. In the previous example, the group's task involved the discussion of a particularly difficult case, one which challenged the competency of the medical and nursing staff and thus, one they preferred not to have to deal with. They found Jane's off-target commentary helpful in letting them avoid what they feared. To help them realize their denial and avoidance, the leader confronted them directly: e.g., "I think that this group is not sure about how to deal with this case. It's the kind of challenge that makes us aware of our own uncertainties as health professionals and so we prefer to avoid discussing it. We joke; we laugh nervously; we let Jane lead us into digressions. I feel that in pointing this out, I'm violating an implicit understanding that we not openly deal with this troublesome case. But I believe that this is a hurdle that we must overcome."

Confrontation and Support. The combination of *confrontation and support* can be one of the most effective change-inducing feedback techniques. Without confrontation—that is, without introducing some doubt, tension, or challenge into the system—there is little likelihood of change. And yet, without a supportive climate to reassure and build confidence, confrontation is likely to result in defensiveness rather than in learning. The leader who would only confront is thereby not likely to be helpful in permitting groups or individuals to learn from their behavior; defensiveness results. Likewise, the leader who is only supportive, who never introduces challenges that produce growth and that drive us to reevaluate our existing ways of behaving, is not likely to help the group or its members move forward as far as they might. The combination of confrontation and support is an important set of techniques for the leader who serves processing functions.

Advice and Suggestions

It almost goes without saying that one type of leadership intervention involves offering advice or suggestions to individuals or the group. The leader may have greater expertise and knowledge than members or may have a perspective on events that members do not have. Feedback that involves advice or suggestions can be helpful. It must be remembered, however, that we are talking about suggestions and advice and not directives. The goal is not to have members simply follow the leader's suggestions without subjecting them to critical evaluation; rather, it is to provide information that members or individuals can use once they have critically examined and evaluated it.

Summarizing

A team at a large urban hospital was observed at several of its meetings. The observer noted that the material at each meeting was brought up over and over again without any apparent resolution. She also noted that there were no summaries provided at the conclusion of any meeting, nor did the leader prepare a summary statement of the staff's still unresolved issues to open the next meeting. At her request, the team voted to take turns in summarizing each meeting before they ended and in preparing and presenting a listing of unresolved issues at the opening of their next meeting. As a result, the team members felt less frustrated; they were now able to make decisions which they could readily implement.

One of the most useful techniques of processing either individual or group behavior involves putting things together in a summary fashion. In doing this, the leader takes a range of behaviors over some period of time, and organizes and summarizes them for the group. Or, as in the example, the leader may ask the group to engage in its own summarization of what has taken place during a certain period. In either case, the goal of this intervention technique is to place an organized, summary statement of its immediately past action before the group.

For example, the leader can suggest that it will be helpful for the group to spend the last five minutes of its meeting reviewing and summarizing the meeting. The leader may then undertake this review and summary or may have members reconstruct the meeting. This reconstruction can focus on decisions that were made, problems that were confronted, issues still before the group that must be considered for the next meeting, and so forth. In the rush of a day's work and in our interests to get our job done, we often forget how useful it can be simply to pause and review where we have just been, what we have just done, and where we plan to head in our next discussion.

Furthermore, in order to summarize, we must organize our recollections of events just past. In the very process of organizing, we may become aware of things that we had not otherwise considered; we may see relationships among events that we would otherwise have ignored. In other words, the very process of attempting to provide a summary for a meeting can offer new insights and new perspectives on things that have already taken place.

Clarification

So much human communication gets distorted and confused in its movement between the transmitter and receiver that an extremely useful leadership function can be served by having either the leader or members directly clarify what has been said. The goal of this intervention is to check on the meanings of the interaction and communication. Leaders, for example, may ask members to clarify their remarks: e.g., "I'm not certain just what you meant when you stated that you find John's analysis of the case in error. Could you tell us what you mean?"

Or, they may attempt their own clarification: e.g., "What I heard you saying is that you disagree with John's analysis of the case. Is that correct?"

Through clarification, the leader hopes to help the group better understand itself and its communications. In recognition of the often needlessly confusing consequences of misunderstandings, the leader's aim is to help clarify communications that could be misunderstood before members can react to the misunderstandings. There is enough difficulty resulting from real conflicts of interest and clashes of different value systems. This is substantive conflict that a group should confront and work on. Needless conflict, however, is based on faulty communication in transmission or reception. Through clarifying interventions, the leader hopes to minimize the detrimental impact of these kinds of needless and nonsubstantive conflicts.

For example, John and Bill basically agree in what they are saying but fail to hear and to understand each other. By clarifying what has been said, the leader hopes to make it possible for them to see that they are really agreeing. By asking members to clarify what they mean (e.g., "I'm not sure I understand what you just said or meant") and by taking the role of clarifier (e.g., "This is what I hear you saying . . ."), the leader intervenes to facilitate more accurate communication within the group.

Probing and Questioning

Probing and questioning are techniques that trained interviewers learn. Through these methods the respondent is pressed for more information, more material, so that a better understanding or a deeper insight is made possible. Probing and questioning are useful process interventions in group leadership. The leader may probe by directly asking a question: e.g., "You just said that Dr. Williams' approach is something that you find helpful. Could you tell us more about what in his technique you find valuable?" The probe might take a less direct form: e.g., "A new technique?" In this latter example, often the repetition of the last few comments made by a member will serve to trigger a continuation of the member's commentary.

Through probing and questioning the leader hopes to help members generate more material concerning their ideas and opinions. It is not unusual for members simply to state an opinion or viewpoint and leave it at that. This provides little for others to work with; and so the leader may use probing and questioning to get more material out before the group to consider and to evaluate. For example, a member might say in response to another's comments: "No, I don't think that's a good idea." That statement may be made with such finality that there is little that the group can do other than to go on to another member or another issue. But the perceptive leader might probe and question in order to turn that final period into a comma: e.g., "I wish you could tell us more about your own thoughts on this matter; it would be helpful for us to hear more from you."

A *Caution.* Probing by an inexperienced leader can backfire and produce high anxiety in a group or in a member. Improperly done, probing and questioning can make people feel they are being "grilled" or challenged. The idea behind a probe is to help persons say more fully what they know and wish to share; a probe should usually not be used to force people to disclose things that they wish to keep secret; nor should questions be used improperly to make people feel stupid or incompetent. These are some of the pitfalls of probing that the inexperienced leader may inadvertently implement.

A *Guide to Better Probing.* Given some of the problems that improper probing can produce, it is helpful for the leader to use this type of intervention with caution. When questioning and probing are employed there are certain helpful guides for handling the situation. For example, one way of getting more from the speaker is simply to say, "Could you expand a bit further on what you've just said?" This invites more information and gives the person freedom to say no or to go on. When we next consider the technique called repetition, we will note another way to probe for more material without grilling the person. For example, the leader can simply repeat the last few words of the speaker:

SPEAKER: I'm not sure that we should pursue this matter any further.

LEADER: You're not sure about pursuing it?

SPEAKER: Well, there is just one more thing I'd like to talk about here.

Basically, the intent of the probing and questioning technique is to help group members develop and expand on something they are saying. The ideal is to help them do this when they are *ready* to, and about a matter or topic they are *willing* to examine further. Probing is not intended to push people to do something they don't want or aren't ready to do. Probing and questioning, in the hands of the experienced group leader, are more like *invitations* to continue.

Repeating, Paraphrasing, Highlighting

Strictly speaking, repeating, paraphrasing, and highlighting are not different techniques as much as they are components of several of the preceding interventions. They offer the leader a more complete repertoire of process interventions that help provide feedback. The simple act of repeating often facilitates communication among group members. The leader simply repeats back what he or she has heard; this can serve to correct inaccurate communication or emphasize accurate communication.

In the example we used to examine probing, we saw how the repetition of the speaker's words (e.g., "You're not sure about pursuing it?") were helpful in allowing the speaker to decide on the direction of the conversation and to continue or to stop. One of the problems that less experienced leaders often run into is the tendency to lose the speaker's thoughts and intent by placing their own meaning onto it. Thus the leader, not the speaker, decides on the direction of the conversation and we learn more about the leader's concerns than the member's. For example:

MEMBER: I'm not sure that we should pursue this project.

LEADER: Are you afraid that we'd run into the same difficulty here as on our last case?

MEMBER: No, I hadn't thought of that; but now that you mention it, perhaps . . .

What has happened here is that the leader has implanted a doubt or anxiety (one that may well be her own) and has lost the member's own thoughts. Repetition can help avoid or at least minimize that possibility:

MEMBER: I'm not sure that we should pursue this project.

LEADER: You're not sure that we should pursue this project?

MEMBER: That's right. I think it is very foolish of us to think that with our small numbers and lack of facilities we can bring about such a large change as we've proposed.

Note how the repetition has brought the member's own thoughts to light without the improper interposition of the leader's particular worries.

In paraphrasing, the leader hopes to clarify matters by repeating what has been said, but as a paraphrase rather than as a direct repetition. For example, a member might say, "I'm not sure just how we should go about dealing with Mrs. French's family; sometimes I think we'd be better off if we could deal with her and leave her family out of the picture entirely." A paraphrase might take this form: "You're puzzled about what we should do with Mrs. French's family." The purpose of this paraphrase is to *highlight* what the leader senses to be the main thrust of the member's comments. In this way, the group can focus on the main issue and not get overly involved in side issues. At the same time, when the leader's perception of the important element in the member's communication is highlighted, the member can respond with agreement or disagreement. In either case, there has been clarification; communication can flow more accurately within the group.

We should note that in paraphrasing or in highlighting, the leader is offering his or her version of what has been said. This is less likely with repetition. The more the paraphrase or the highlight is removed from what has been said, the more it becomes like an interpretation. We mention this not to discourage leaders from paraphrasing or highlighting, but to caution them that in some cases they are beginning to walk on the territory of interpretation and analysis.

Reflection

In reflecting, the leader focuses the attention of the individual or the group on the important feelings that are being communicated or on the behaviors that are taking place. Thus there are two related, though distinct, types of reflection: of feelings and of behaviors. We will examine each of these.

Reflection of Feelings. An example will help our understanding of the use of reflection of feelings:

MEMBER: I've been working here for many, many years and I think that I know pretty much about proper procedures and things like that. I'm getting tired of hearing from those new, young, fresh-from-college types about the right and proper way we should be doing things around here.

The leader might reflect back to this member and to the others in the group what feelings he or she thinks are being conveyed:

LEADER: You sound upset and annoyed with these young people.

In this type of intervention, the leader orients the members to the feelings that lie behind the content of the person's remarks. In this way, that person is allowed to deal with these feelings directly instead of passing them by as though they did not exist. For example, without the leader's intervention, the response to those comments might have been: "Well, we must get on with our main task today." Other members might avoid dealing with the feelings that lie behind the remarks. The leader, sensing that these feelings are important for the group to consider before continuing, uses reflection as a technique to bring the feelings to the focus of the group.

It need not only be an individual's feelings that are reflected, however; the leader may reflect feelings that are more generally shared, though unstated, among the group.

> A nurse is working with a parent group in the community that is concerned with issues of sexuality. She is introducing her lecture on the anatomy and physiology of male and female sexual functioning and notices that there is much giggling and uneasiness among group members.

The nurse can either continue with her lecture, completely ignoring the parents' uneasiness, or she can intervene at this point by reflecting their feelings to them: e.g., "I sense that many of you are made anxious by this discussion. Perhaps this is something we should talk about before I continue with the lecture itself."

In the reflection of feelings, the leader searches behind the content of communications and responds to the feelings that are being conveyed either by *what* is said or by *how* it is said. Members may be talking about matters that on the surface seem to be nonemotional in content. The leader, however, notices some nonverbal behavior that suggests that there are strong feelings behind the mask of apparently neutral content. Lou says to Sam, in an apparently calm manner, "What you say is interesting, but I'm not sure that I can agree fully with you about it." The leader may notice that there is anger being communicated nonverbally: e.g., Lou's face tightens, her hands form a fist, she leans forward in an aggressive stance. These tell the leader about Lou's feelings. The leader then reflects these feelings: e.g., "I sense that you are very angry with Sam." These feelings can now become a focus for consideration.

Reflection of Behavior. In reflecting individual or group *behavior*, the leader engages in less interpretation than is usually involved when reflecting feelings. Thus, for example, the nurse working with the parent group might simply have reflected to them the fact that they are giggling and stirring about restlessly in their chairs. She may have then asked them what this could mean. The reflection of behavior involves informing the members what behavior the leader sees them carrying out: this will include nonverbal behavior of which the member may be aware or unaware (e.g., "I notice much restless moving about in the chairs"). It will also include verbal behaviors, as in the following example:

MEMBER: I'm not sure what is expected of me around here; you old-timers seem to know what is going on; I'm still wet behind the ears; you old hands surely have better skills than I do; I'm fresh from college.

LEADER: I've noticed the words you use to describe yourself and the words you use to describe the others. They are all "old timers" and "old hands" and you're "still wet behind the ears." Could you tell us what you are feeling about being in this group?

As this example indicates, the leader has reflected back the member's actual *behavior* to him—in this case, the words he used in describing or explaining something. The leader, however, could also have reflected back the member's *feelings* to him: e.g., "You sound upset and anxious with your status as a new person in a group of experienced people."

Notice, however, that to reflect feelings requires greater degree of interpretation than to reflect behaviors. The leader must be sensitive to this important distinction. Telling members what you see them doing or hear them saying is different than telling them what feelings you *think* they are expressing by what they are doing and saying. The former is more directly observational; the latter more interpretative and inferential. We are suggesting that the reflection of feelings should be done with great care and with a genuine openness to being incorrect.

Interpretation and Analysis

Interpretative interventions go several steps beyond sheer observation of individual or group behavior. The observations that the leader makes are placed within a theoretical context that gives them meaning; it is this meaning that is then fed back to the group or individual. The following is a brief illustration of interpretation as distinct from several of the other techniques we have considered:

GROUP MEMBER: I feel terrible about missing so many group meetings. (He speaks softly and hesitantly; his head is lowered; his brow is knitted; he bites his lips and wrings his hands.)

LEADER PARAPHRASING: Yes, you have missed several meetings.

LEADER REPEATING: You feel terrible about having missed so many meetings?

LEADER PROBING: Frankly, I was puzzled about your behavior. Why did you miss so many meetings?

LEADER REFLECTING FEELINGS: You sound rather upset and worried.

LEADER REFLECTING BEHAVIOR: While telling us this, your face is lowered, your brow is tightly knit, you are rubbing your hands together, and your voice is soft and hesitant. How are you feeling?

LEADER CONFRONTING: It seems to me that having missed so many meetings must make it difficult for you to participate actively in this group. Just what do you plan to do about it?

LEADER INTERPRETING: I am beginning to wonder about why you have missed so many of our meetings or if there is a pattern to your absences. Although I'm not sure, I wonder if you are asking us to pay more attention to you but are asking this in a way that actually works to your disadvantage?

(Schulman, 1974 offers a similar example.)

The leader's interpretation takes the observation of several absences and looks for some underlying pattern that gives meaning to that behavior. The meaning comes from locating the behavior in a larger theoretical context; that is, a particular behavior is rendered meaningful by virtue of its fitting into a theory. This is one reason why leaders must have clear understanding of theory in order to be able to intervene with interpretive or analytic comments.

In the example, the interpretation suggests that the member, for some reason, has need for more attention from the group and has used a nonproductive manner of seeking that attention, as if to say: "You'll really notice me when I'm not here." As the leader notes, excessive absence produces just the opposite effect; the member becomes even more distanced from the group and receives less and less attention.

The interpretive intervention is designed to help the member see his behavior from a new perspective. The hope is that this new view will help him gain better conscious control over his behavior and effect a change in it. That is, if the member really wants more attention, he must see that absences are not an effective way to get it. We leave out of this consideration the reasons why so much attention is needed; rather, we focus on the behavior and one level of interpretation; in this case, the aim is to help the person see that his goals are not being achieved by that particular behavior.

Let us take another example. Fran is a member who frequently says that she wants to be accepted and liked by others in her group. And yet, when she interacts with others, she continually interrupts them, cuts them off in mid-sentence, only rarely supports and agrees with them, and in any number of other ways seems to reject the very persons she says she wants to have accept her. The leader may choose to make an interpretive intervention:

> Fran—I've heard you say on several occasions that you are concerned about being liked and accepted by this group. And yet, I watch your behavior and notice that you tend to be abrupt, to interrupt others, to be overly critical of their comments, rarely to support or agree with them. You seem to me to act in ways that will not get others to like you or accept you. This leads me to wonder why you're doing this. I wonder if perhaps you so fear being rejected that you reject others before they have a chance either to accept or to reject you?

There are several features of this interpretation that need to be noted.

1. It summarizes Fran's past behavior and presents this summary to her. Thus it is an interpretation that is rooted to concrete behaviors. This helps Fran better see what there is about her and her behavior that can be corrected if she chooses or is able to do so.

2. It offers an analysis of Fran's behavior and what may be a deeper reason or meaning for it. In this case, the analysis is provided by a theoretical perspective that suggests that acceptance/rejection is an important issue for all of us; that, in fear of being rejected by others, some of us act to reject these others first. In this way we avoid discovering whether or not we are worthy of acceptance by creating our own conclusion.

3. This level of interpretation, though several steps removed from our observations, is not as deep an analysis as we could make. That is, the leader does not seek to probe much further beneath the surface to understand the whys and wherefores of Fran's fear of rejection or why she rejects before she is rejected.

The leader does not probe in order to understand some of the deeper bases for Fran's lack of self-esteem. The leader is content, rather, to focus on the actual behavior and some of its immediate consequences. We are not dealing with therapy or therapy groups in which interpretations that uncover more material at deeper levels of meaning may be necessary and important. In most groups, however, it is necessary to analyze in a way that will help members see the effects of their behavior; this lets them work to remedy those effects even though we and they may never attempt to get at the deeper causes that may persist. In the example, Fran can use the leader's interpretation to observe how her manner of interacting with others thwarts her gaining the acceptance she claims she so desperately wants. Thus, Fran can see that one of the consequences of her behavior is that it prevents her being accepted by others.

Group-Level Interpretations. Interpretations can also be made at the group level. For example, a consultant is called in to help a group diagnose and evaluate its difficulties. He observes that the group is led by a rather directive and autocratic leader; members fail to express any anger and resentment toward this leader. The consultant notices, however, that one member of the group seems to be the butt of jokes and criticisms, and is generally picked on excessively: i.e., this person's behavior does not seem to warrant his receiving the kind of treatment that he gets. From the consultant's perspective, this member appears to be the group's scapegoat, receiving all the angry and resentful feelings that members have toward their leader which they fear to express directly and openly.

The consultant decides to confront the group with this interpretation: "I've observed your meeting for some time now and have some impressions that I would like to share with you. First, I've noticed that Jerry seems to be the butt of much anger and resentment. As I watch his behavior, however, I have difficulty in seeing just what he's done to deserve all this anger. I wonder if perhaps there is some resentment that members have toward John, the group leader, that they are fearful of expressing and so have chosen Jerry as their scapegoat?"

There is no magic in this interpretive formulation. The members may respond with anger at the consultant, accusing him of coming in to mess up their otherwise happy group. The group leader may feel very threatened, not only by the consultant's presence in a challenging role but also by his interpretive remarks and their implication about his leadership style. Members may feel threatened by now having to consider directly and openly their hostilities toward their leader rather than continuing to use the faithful scapegoat, Jerry. They may now make the consultant their scapegoat. On the other hand, it is possible that the time is ripe for the group members to openly explore their behavior and that the consultant's interpretive intervention was just the catalyst they needed.

Listening

Good and attentive listening is perhaps one of the most important and critical processing approaches for leaders. Groups often become arenas for members simply to speak their piece without listening or responding to others. The process thus becomes somewhat like the parallel play of children, a loosely connected chaining of talkers none of whom pays attention to the others or to do more than minimally respond to others. The function of the leader as a listener can be critical.

In the first place, a listening leader gives members an attentive audience to whom they can address their remarks; it provides them someone who is responsive to what they say when no one else might be.

In the second place, the attentive, listening leader can help shape group process by *modeling* a desirable form of behavior. When leaders not only listen attentively with an aim to truly understanding what is being said and also act in ways that demonstrate this responsiveness—e.g., by responding appropriately to members' comments rather than by simply going off on their own track as others tend to do—then members can see the possibilities for their behaving in a similarly attentive and responsive manner.

Finally, an attentive and responsive listener can help speakers sharpen their own thinking and understanding. We all get sloppy in our speech and logic when we sense that no one is really listening or trying to understand us anyway. But the realization that there is someone who is both listening and trying to understand can force us to become more aware of just what we are saying. Although this may be somewhat inhibiting at first, in time listening can be highly instructive to members, especially when they make a concerted effort not only to talk in more communicative ways but also to become better listeners themselves.

Timing

If a cookbook of interpersonal skills could be written, surely it would specify precisely the proper timing for leader interventions. However, no serious student of group process would write a cookbook; it is just too complex a subject. Timing is the most critical and difficult lesson of all to learn. Regardless of the technique employed, the leader must choose intelligently and carefully the timing of any intervention. To intervene too soon by confronting or interpreting may elicit defensiveness. On the other hand, to let matters go and be allowed to build up pressure when they should have been dealt with earlier is not helpful either.

In other words, the leader might wish to "strike while the iron is hot" because "there is no better time than the present" or might properly sense that "silence is golden" and "discretion is the better part of valor." Proper timing involves a very sensitive assessment of the group and its situation. There are no hard and fast rules for definitive guidance. Experience can be an excellent teacher. In general, however, it is wise first to facilitate the creation of a supportive climate, one within which members feel secure enough with themselves and their leader to take some risks. The leader must explore the group's process *before* intervening with confrontation or interpretation.

Basically, the leader must remember that the goal is to help the group process its ongoing behavior so that members may work together more effectively. The leader must evaluate timing in terms of whether or not an intervention at a particular point will help the group better achieve its goals.

One of the best ways of learning about timing is to venture forth and try. Ask the group: "Are my comments timed to be as helpful as they might be?" Make a trial intervention. If there are loud denials or if people ignore you completely, then perhaps your timing is off. Wait and try again later.

Obviously, a group that is meeting only once must be dealt with differently than a group that meets on a continuing basis. The former cannot tolerate much process intervention; its members do not have the time to deal with complex interpretations, challenging confrontations, or reflections of feelings. A leader who intervenes to point out a process that must be worked on and evaluated by the group must realize that time is needed to do this work. It is poor and inappropriate timing therefore to intervene with process-type comments when there is no time or opportunity for members to follow up and evaluate what new doors and perspectives the leader has opened.

Time is needed to work on material that process interventions bring to light. Thus to intervene late in a session may be a poor idea—a summary might be more helpful at such a point. Likewise, just after a meeting has begun can be a bad time to interpret and to analyze, unless members have a past history of working effectively together in processing their ongoing actions.

RESISTANCE AND PROCESSING

Dr. Romero is the director of one of the hospital's units. He sets aside a half-hour each week for the staff members to "process" (his term) their own interpersonal material. At 2 P.M. sharp each Wednesday, after the staff has convened, he says, "Well, what are our concerns this week?" The staff has great resistance to this processing of their own relationships. It is a new idea to most of them; it is frightening. For almost five months they have talked about how hard it is to do. A new member has joined the staff. She becomes quite angry during these sessions and keeps saying, "You people don't dare examine your own relationships as staff members or your feelings about Dr. Romero." The resistance does not decrease. But gradually, as tensions on the unit increase—primarily because administrative pressures are increasing and the severity of patients' illness is proving disturbing to most of the staff—they begin to test the idea of sharing. They begin to examine their relationship as staff members and note that their tensions, especially those from external sources (e.g., administration and patients) begin to diminish as they do this. The atmosphere on the entire unit begins to clear and lighten. Their resistance has faded considerably and they now almost eagerly await those weekly sessions.

As the example suggests, processing as a leadership function is by no means heartily accepted either by leaders or by group members. There are many bases for resistance to the processing function. It will help us to examine four of these: (1) the difficulty in perceiving one's self behaving; (2) polite norms that shy away from examining ongoing behavior; (3) power plays and the tactics of winning that lead people to suspect the motives of those who would process and provide feedback; (4) the fear of looking foolish, acting inappropriately, or appearing weak.

Perceiving Ongoing Behavior

We should really not consider this first point as much a matter of resistance as a matter of a basic human difficulty. We cannot simultaneously behave and see ourselves behaving. To try to become conscious of ourselves behaving disrupts our performance. For example, we can read and we can write; but if we focus our attention on the actual process by which our reading or writing is taking place, it disrupts the reading or writing. However, we are able to stop and reflect back on what we have done; or we can use others as sources of information for our own activitiy.

Paradoxically, we are directly in touch with others at the moment of their behaving but are in touch with ourselves only *after* we have behaved (Schutz, 1970–1971). We see others directly and immediately and ourselves reflectively. We need those others, therefore, to keep us informed about our behavior and its effects. Their feedback plays a critical role in informing us about ourselves. Naturally, we can pause and reflect back on our own actions and thereby supply our own feedback. Or, as several efforts have demonstrated (e.g., Storms, 1973), we can use videotape to play back our own actions, giving us an observer's view of ourselves; but this is the kind of view we cannot obtain without a device such as a video recorder.

Whether we use others to give us feedback, pause and reflect on our own actions, or use some mechanical recording device, in all cases we need information about our actions in order to evaluate and adjust. We need feedback before we can function more effectively and learn how to improve the next time around. Groups are in a similar position. Members get so caught up in developing their own points of view that they cannot see what is going on or how their behavior contributes to the group's getting bogged down in detail when it needs to take stock of itself.

The difficulties we have in seeing ourselves behaving and interacting with others makes adjustment in our performances, and hence our learning, a real problem. We must openly court feedback from others, or pause frequently to reflect on ourselves, in order to modify our actions in light of the condequences they produce.

Social Norms

As several analysts have noted (e.g., Argyris, 1976; Yalom, 1975), it is not polite to process another person's behavior. Parents do it with their children, commenting on the ways they are behaving and the consequences of behaving in those ways: "You are shouting now; why are you so angry?" "Don't talk to me like that!" When adults call attention to these matters, we feel they are behaving impolitely. And yet, it is just this kind of normative violation that is required to fulfill the leadership function of processing. There cannot be any processing for a group unless people, both leaders and members, are willing to drop some of the polite norms that discourage their focusing on and reviewing ongoing behavior.

The typical response, however, when norms have been violated is to try to normalize the situation again. If one person processes what she believes is taking place, others may respond by angrily denying that anything is taking place other than what we have all seen or heard; or that the person doing the processing must be crazy; or they might try to ignore it all together and continue as though nothing had happened.

NURSE ASH: Doctor Sells, I have the feeling that whenever you give me an order you do so with a kind of arrogance that says to me that either you are insecure about me or frightened of me, or something like that.

DR. SELLS: I'm sure I don't know what you're talking about. Anyway, what does it matter? Your job is clear. Follow precisely what I say.

NURSE ASH: It's not that. I'm not questioning your authority; I'm not even challenging your orders. I was just wondering if you felt some need to put me down by acting so arrogantly whenever you address me.

DR. SELLS: That's stupid. Why would I want to do something like that! Now, let's get back to our rounds.

There are several important implications of the normative view of resistance. A leader must play an active part in helping create new norms. Or, the leader must support those members who are more willing than others to engage in processing, who are willing to violate norms that forbid its usage. Basically, the leader must help create an atmosphere in which processing and feedback are part of the normal and routine life of the group. A leader who would simply process without having created a normative climate for it or helping to explain its usefulness is simply asking for trouble, resistance, and rejection.

One way for the leader to help break down the resistant old norms and facilitate the emergence of norms that are most hospitable to processing is for the leader to ask for feedback about his or her own behavior. This can also help clear the way for others to engage in similar activities. It also makes the leader appear more human, vulnerable, and approachable.

Social Power

Unfortunately, processing and feedback are too often used as weapons of battle than as techniques for serious group self-evaluation. Many people process the behavior of others as a way to get back at them, to demean them, to put them down, to hurt them, to put them in their place, to score points, to win, or whatever. Understanding and self-correction are not the goal of this kind of processing; winning is.

For this reason people suspect processing; it makes the one processed more vulnerable and thereby triggers defenses. When we report people's behavior back to them, they tend not to be open and receptive to hearing about it; rather, they almost instinctively put up defenses, to deny it, to argue about it, or better still to pick on a piece of *our* behavior and cast it back quickly to put us off our guard. Processing in the name of winning and of garnering more power is not helpful to group interaction. However, processing that equalizes the vulnerability, that opens up the lines of communication, is useful. Thus leaders who court feedback on their own behavior make themselves more vulnerable; this now equalizes the vulnerability that members tend to experience and so can reduce resistance.

The motivations behind processing, therefore, must be clear in the minds of those who do it. If they are out to prove a point—their own, or make a point—their own, or score a point—their own, or demonstrate how perceptive and insightful they are, then they are not processing in the service of accomplishing effective group functioning. Their aims are not to help a group evaluate its course and its alternatives, but rather to demonstrate something about themselves and their relationships to others. They use processing as a weapon to gain or to maintain power over others.

Stated in another way, one who processes must be open to being processed. One cannot hope to feed information back into a group without thereby becoming a part of that group's process. The contributor creates a position of vulnerability for himself or herself within the group. One cannot process as a spectator, as though casting the first stone and then rushing away; rather, one must process from inside and thereby become as vulnerable as everyone else. It is no wonder, then, that so many group leaders shy away from this kind of bilateral engagement, preferring to exercise their unilateral control and thereby avoid being vulnerable.

The beneficial function of processing requires the processor to be processed as well. The leader who asks the group to stop and evaluate itself must remember that he or she thereby is open to evaluation as well. It is not simply that the leader, from outside or on high, says, "You take a look at where you are and where you are going." From within the group, the leader says, "Let us take a look at ourselves, where we have been and where we are going. And let us look at the kind of leadership I am providing and how this too can be improved."

Fear

Because processing behavior places the leader and members on a more equal standing, opening up their relationship to examination and evaluation, many leaders, as we have noted, shy away from its use. They choose a more autocratic style and avoid any hints at processing, unless they see a way for it to be used unilaterally toward their own ends. But there is another leader-based resistance to processing: fear.

Argyris (1976) captures this fear perfectly in his discussion of a group of business executives who finally learned the perceptual and interpersonal skills of processing and became proficient in its use but who still were fearful of using it back home in their organizations. When probed about their reasons for this fear, it was discovered that they felt their subordinates would think them foolish, inappropriate, or weak as leaders. Quite a strong set of reasons not to put into practice the excellent leadership skills that they had just learned!

The terrible trio—foolish, inappropriate, and weak—consisted of precisely the feelings they had had when first entering the training course in which they learned how to engage in the processing functions of leadership. Their first sessions were spent in commenting on the foolishness of the business executive who asks others to reflect on their behavior with him; on the inappropriateness of this; of the weakness and vulnerability that it suggested. After all, only a weak leader would do anything other than dominate and lead with great confidence and self-assurance.

These fears are difficult to overcome; in fact, it is only through the use of processing that group leaders begin to experience its advantages and to experience themselves as stronger through its use and as weaker without.

Reflect for a moment on the possibility of leaders who dominate the discussion and direct others toward their ends vs. leaders who confidently open up their group and their leadership to frequent self-examination. Who are the more foolish, less appropriate, and weaker of the two? We suspect the self-confidence of leaders who would never examine their practice, who would never reflect with their group on its process, who would never wish to evaluate their own or their group's actions.

THE LIMITS OF LEADERSHIP

We have been examining group leadership in this and the preceding chapter. It is possible to come away supposing that the entire story of a group lies entirely in the hands of the leader. To be sure, good leadership is essential; but it is only part of the total picture. There are definite limits to leadership that no amount of skill and training can help overcome.

In a rather monumental research effort evaluating different types of therapy-group leadership, Lieberman, Yalom, and Miles (1973) suggested that a leader's behaviors and style cannot overcome strongly held group norms that oppose them. Leaders who would impose their style on a group composed of persons who, for whatever reasons, have created a set of norms that ran counter to that style, could hardly be successful in leading that group. To be sure, over a long period of time and hard work together, member norms might change to accommodate the leader's preferences. But in the context of most groups, the leader must work within the limits defined by the groups norms.

Leaders can and do play a significant role in shaping those norms. Three possibilities exist for the leader. First, it is important for a leader to enter early into affecting the norms the group will evolve. A leader who seeks to be more democratic and to build upon the processing function, for example, must work early to help members learn and understand this style. To wait too long might result in the formation of group norms that are antithetical to a democratic processing style. Second, leaders can build upon the diversity of members' own expectations regarding their group and its proper functioning; they can support a set of norms that are more congruent with their style and goals. Finally, leaders can play an influential role in setting norms in areas of ambiguity, where members' expectations are unclear and the gentle nudge of leadership is advice well heeded by the members.

But the limits are there. Members bring with them sets of expectations and background experiences that play a significant role in the kinds of norms that the group will develop; these create the boundaries within which the leader may function. A group that defines narrow boundaries will strongly limit the leader's ability to work outside those boundaries. The burden then does not lie entirely on the leader's shoulders. Leaders are important and their skills essential; but group norms create limits within which leaders must function.

We are reminded of a very process-oriented, democratic leader who was asked to lead a discussion group of very highly structured, deferent persons. These members arrived with a strong set of expectations regarding proper leader and member behavior. In their view, the leader was to lead, to direct, to command; members were to follow and to work within the structure the leader set down.

Each attempt this leader made to help the group set its own agenda was met with a passive, "You tell us what you want us to do." She processed these remarks by noting, "You seem to be highly concerned with what I want you to do; but I really want you to discover first what *you* are interested in doing and want to do." Members smiled and said, "You are right, we *want* you to tell us what we should be doing."

In this particular group, there were no members with a differing point of view regarding proper leader behavior. And try as she would to engage them in dialogue to explore their own desires, it always returned to the one point, "We'll do whatever you want us to do." The limits of this leadership were clear; the boundaries of this group were very narrow and stringent, tolerating no deviation. Leadership is a two-way street. Members play a significant role in the style of leadership that will evolve and be useful for their group.

SUMMARY AND CONCLUSIONS

The functions of leadership require careful study and understanding of all the chapters that have preceded this one and a consideration of the material in the remaining chapter. Chapters artificially segment and isolate the kinds of knowledge and skills that must be woven together if one is to work effectively as a group leader or as a helpful and effective group member.

Table 11–1 provides a useful summary of the various types of leader interventions that we have covered in this chapter. The table indicates both the types that we have discussed and the important goals and functions each type is said to serve.

Table 11–1. A Summary of Leader Interventions

Type of Intervention	Goals of Intervention
Support	Provides supportive climate for expressing ideas and opinions, including unpopular or unusual points of view.
	Facilitates members continuing with their ongoing behavior.
	Helps reinforce positive forms of behavior.
	Creates a climate in which silent members may feel secure enough to participate.
Confrontation	Aids in growth and development; helps unfreeze members from being stuck in one mode of functioning.
	Helps reduce some forms of disruptive behavior.
	Helps members deal more openly and directly with each other.
Advice and Suggestions	Shares expertise, offers new perspectives.
	Helps focus group on its task and goals.
Summarizing	Helps keep group on its task by reviewing past actions and by setting agenda for future sessions.
	Brings to focus still unresolved issues.

Table 11–1. *(Continued)*

Type of Intervention	Goals of Intervention
	Organizes past in ways that help clarify; brings into focus themes and patterns of interaction.
Clarifying	Helps reduce distortion in communication.
	Facilitates focus on substantive issues rather than allowing members to be side-tracked into misunderstandings.
Probing and Questioning	Helps expand a point that may have been left incomplete.
	Gets at more extensive and wider range of information.
	Invites members to explore their ideas in greater detail.
Repeating, Paraphrasing, and Highlighting	Helps members continue with their ongoing behavior; invites further exploration and examination of what is being said.
	Clarifies and helps focus on the specific, important, or key aspect of a communication.
	Sharpens members' understanding of what is being said or done.
Reflecting: Feelings	Orients members to the feelings that may lie behind what is being said or done.
	Helps members deal with issues they might otherwise avoid or miss.
Reflecting: Behavior	Gives members the opportunity to see how their behavior appears to others and to see and evaluate its consequences.
	Helps members to understand others' perceptions and responses to them.
Interpretation and Analysis	Renders behavior meaningful by locating it in a larger context in which a causal explanation is provided.

Table 11–1. *(Continued)*

Type of Intervention	*Goals of Intervention*
	Helps members understand both the likely bases of their behavior and its meaning.
	Summarizes a pattern of behavior and provides a useful way of examining it and working to modify it through the insights gained.
Listening	Provides an attentive and responsive audience for those who participate.
	Models a helpful way for members to relate to one another; gives a feeling of sharing and mutual concern.
	Helps members sharpen their own ideas and thinking as they realize that indeed others are listening and concerned about what they are saying.

12

How to Deal with Typical Group Problems: An Intervention Model

The health professional who leads groups usually has many "how-to" questions about issues encountered in most groups. In this final chapter, we will examine seven issues that group leaders often confront:

1. Dealing with the member who dominates or monopolizes the discussion
2. Dealing with the silent member or the apathetic-silent group
3. Dealing with emotional outbursts such as anger or crying
4. Dealing with group conflict
5. Dealing with normative deviance, with behaviors that violate group norms and expectations for proper member behavior
6. Dealing with the issues involved in beginning a group
7. Dealing with the issues involved in ending or terminating a group.

This chapter, by itself, without careful consideration of the material in the preceding chapters, can have an excessively mechanical quality to it. As with most skilled professional activities, technical competence, while important, does not comprise the entire picture that is necessary for effective leadership. This chapter builds upon the work of the preceding chapters and assumes a general familiarity and understanding on the part of the reader, of that work. Its "cookbook" appearance is deceptive. One cannot simply follow a recipe for group intervention techniques and get from here to there.

It is especially important for the practitioner to recognize that subtle interpersonal factors involving concern and empathy are as important for the group leader as the skills with which this chapter primarily deals. Likewise, a solid grounding in group process theory is prerequisite to effective leadership. Technical skills for intervention strategies must be built upon this solid foundation of knowledge and a genuine concern for one's group and its members.

A GENERAL MODEL OF INTERVENTION

The first matter at hand is the introduction of a general intervention model relevant to any questions and answers involving group and interpersonal behavior. The model contains five distinct stages; each requires leaders to engage in a process both before and after their actual intervention in the group. These five stages are summarized in Table 12–1.

As the table indicates, the first task facing the leader involves defining the nature and scope of the problem. This entails weaving together theoretical understanding with behavioral observations in order to develop a diagnosis to guide the intervention strategies that will be used. From the more theoretical side, the leader must be sensitive to what we have termed the underlying issues and accompanying consequences that are typically involved in a particular problem. For example, a single member who dominates a discussion can produce an apathetic and nonproductive group as others withdraw their own involvement and let the dominating member carry the ball. The leader must be sensitive to this aspect of the problem.

By observation we simply mean that any intervention in a group must be based upon observational material. Leaders must first observe individual or group behavior, including the patterns of behavior that occur within a group. Their intervention must not only follow from these observations but as importantly must refer back to the behavioral observations. That is, leaders cannot simply intervene like a bolt out of the blue, no matter how exciting, or full of insight their intervention might be. It is hardly helpful for an individual or group members to accept a leader's thoughtful interventions without hearing as well the observational base for those interventions:

> The leader, John, says to a member, Agnes, "I have noticed that you arrive late to most of our meetings. I have also noticed that the group does not begin officially until you arrive. So, when you are very late, as you

Table 12–1. An Intervention Model

DEFINING THE PROBLEM	
1. ISSUE:	Why is this a problem?
	What are its dimensions and its possibilities for affecting group process?
2. OBSERVATIONS:	What behaviors do I see taking place within the group and its members?
3. DIAGNOSIS:	What does it mean?
	What understanding can I conclude about the behavior from my observations and my grasp of the issues that are involved?
ENTERING THE GROUP PROCESS	
4. INTERVENTION STRATEGIES:	What are some specific techniques that I can use to enter the group's process to affect the problem?
ASSESSING THE EFFECTS	
5. EVALUATION:	What was the effect of my intervention?
	How do I gauge my success or my failure?

have often been, we simply wait around, doing little until your arrival. It is getting to be very wasteful of our time. I think this is something we have to examine and do something about."

The diagnostic stage of the intervention process requires that leaders use direct behavioral observations plus their knowledge of theory to make a tentative diagnosis of the problem at hand. A diagnosis is an inference that connects observational material to some larger body of knowledge (e.g., a theory); diagnoses render that material meaningful and direct toward an intervention strategy.

In the preceding example of the late-arriving member, the leader's diagnosis might be that Agnes' late arrival is a power ploy on her part. She knows that the group does not begin until she arrives; she can thereby demonstrate her power and control over the group by managing her arrival time.

It is important to realize that any diagnosis may be incorrect or at best partially correct. Human behavior is determined in a complex multitude of ways. There is no simple, single one-to-one correspondence between a behavior and a given meaning or diagnostic category. Agnes' lateness undoubtedly has other meanings as well: e.g., she had a long way to come to arrive on time for the group meetings. However, when a behavior *becomes consistent over time*, forming a pattern (e.g., her lateness occurs nearly every time the group meets); and when that pattern has a compelling rationale for one meaning over another (e.g., she arrives late even when meetings have been announced well in advance, when she and others have noted meeting times in their notebooks, when leaving in time to make the meeting is possible at least on several occasions); and finally, when other behaviors are noted that form an overall consistency with the diagnosis so that it is not based merely on one action but rather a matrix of behaviors (e.g., the power interpretation is consistent with Agnes' other behavior in the group: she frequently challenges the leader's authority; she seeks to dominate meetings by talking a great deal; she seems to enjoy having members turn to her for advice), then it would appear that the diagnosis is a reasonable one. Basically, as with any diagnostic process, one is looking for multiple operations that converge upon a given diagnosis and make it more compelling than any alternative.

The intervention stage involves the actions that leaders take, what is said and done to effect group process. In Chapter 11 we examined many of these intervention techniques for group leaders. We will pursue these further in this chapter as specific ways to deal with particular issues and problems facing a group.

Evaluation is a necessary follow-up to intervention. The leader's interest is in checking out and evaluating the consequences of his or her intervention. An evaluation can extend from an attempt to validate his or her own analysis against other members' analyses to an effort to judge whether or not the intervention produced the desired effect: e.g., did the group now deal with Agnes' lateness so that members could use their time more effectively together?

Our discussion of the issues that follow will be organized in terms of this model. For each of the seven problems, we will indicate the dimensions or aspects of the problem, the various kinds of observation that are relevant to recognizing it, the kinds of diagnosis that are likely, several useful interventions, and ways to evaluate the effects of these interventions.

DEALING WITH A MEMBER WHO MONOPOLIZES OR DOMINATES THE GROUP

Issue

For most purposes it is desirable for there to be a relative equality of member participation. Most meetings have time limitations; the monopolization of the conversation by any one member deprives others of their fair share of participation. It is useful to think of participation as a resource or commodity within groups. One person who possesses all of that commodity (e.g., by dominating the conversation) denies others their share of this resource. A sense of injustice tends to develop. The issue facing the leader, therefore (or for that matter, members who feel that they are being denied their share of what usually is a scarce resource), is how to deal with this conversational monopolizer.

This is by no means a trivial matter. Several consequences follow from the presence of a monopolizer in a group. The sense of injustice tends to create bad feelings and anger among members; these can be highly disruptive to the group as a whole. Members' anger and frustration may also be directed toward the group's leader, as though asking, "Why don't you do something to stop that person from monopolizing the discussion!" Thus, leaders who refuse to intervene may find themselves a target of group anger, some of it displaced onto them from the more direct target (the monopolizer) and some more directly concerned with his or her failure to handle this type of disruption. Furthermore, if one person dominates the discussion, the kinds of diversity of viewpoint necessary to make group work effective cannot be realized. There are many important reasons, therefore, for the group leader's intervention.

Observations

One does not need a chart and stopwatch in order to observe some of the behavioral manifestations of monopolization. Some things to look for include: incessant talking, almost compulsive in nature; inability to keep still and to listen; tendency to interrupt others who start to talk; tendency to finish others' thoughts and sentences; frequently tangential and confusing style of talking; a driven quality in which what is said is less important than the sheer fact of saying something. Restlessness and inattentiveness among other group members can also be seen as their response to the monopolizer's domination. Symptoms of frustration and anger, especially deflected toward the leader, can usually be noted among the members.

Diagnosis

At one level of analysis, the compulsive, driven quality of talking may reflect a high level of anxiety. If this diagnosis is tentatively made, then other symptoms of anxiety should be sought. For example, does the person fidget, smoke a lot, move about, show excessive body movements?

Excessive talking can also indicate a strong need for attention. A young child may constantly demand parental attention, especially within a competitive setting in which he or she is vying with other children for the favors of the adults. In a group, the monopolizer may be competing with other group members for the attention, recognition, and approval of the leader.

It would not be surprising to discover that compulsive talkers who monopolize the group's time are not very aware either of their behavior or its consequences. They are too busy behaving (e.g., talking) to pause and observe what they are doing or what effects it may have. The major concern here is not psychotherapy—thus we do not probe deeply into the whys and wherefores of the monopolist's behavior. Rather, the goal is primarily to effect a reasonable behavior change. Therefore, we would diagnose the problem as one requiring an intervention that helps the person (a) see his or her behavior, (b) see its effects on the group, (c) change the behavior to give others an opportunity to participate as well. This last point is important. Our intervention goal is not to completely shut off such people from participating in the group, but rather only to help moderate their participation.

Although we may personally diagnose the person's issue as involving anxiety or need for recognition and approval, we would typically be more concerned with effecting a change in behavior (i.e., reducing their domination of the group) than in probing these underlying dynamics. Therefore, while it may be helpful to interpret some of these possibilities to the individual, it is more often better simply to direct our efforts toward the behavior and its effects on the group.

Interventions

There are several types of interventions that we can use. All of them require that we first interrupt and get the individual to hear us. A simple and direct interruption that may be sufficient in some cases would be, for example, "Thank you very much Jones; I really hate to cut you off right here, but I feel that it is important for us to hear from everyone here. Perhaps we can return to you after others have had a chance to speak their piece." This type of interruption can and should be given in a supportive manner: e.g., "That is a very interesting and a potentially valuable idea; we only have a short time to meet today, however, and I think it best if we move on. Perhaps we can hear others' responses to your ideas."

In the preceding examples, the leader does not make any real effort to help the person see the behavior and its effects on others. If the compulsive monopolizer has been engaging in this kind of behavior for some time (e.g., over several meetings) or if they have not been responsive to a supportive interruption, the leader might then intervene with one or more of the following.

1. *Reflect behavior:* Jones, we are really having trouble hearing from everyone today because you are taking up so much time talking. I wonder if you are aware of this." It would be reasonable at this point for the leader to solicit feedback regarding Jones' behavior from others in the group: "Does anyone else feel this way?"

2. *Interpretation:* Jones, I'm not sure that you are aware that you have talked so much of the time today that hardly anyone else has had a chance. I'm not sure just what it means, but perhaps you're feeling a little anxious about something or concerned with how you come across in this group?" This would be offered as a proposal needing testing. The testing would involve checking with other group members to see if they too feel that Jones is talking excessively and what some of their own interpretations are. In all cases, support is given to Jones to further probe and explore some of the reasons for the behavior.

3. *Reflect group feelings:* Jones, I've noticed that you have been talking a great deal today—so much so, in fact, that few others have been able to participate. I've also noticed myself and maybe many others in the

group getting bored and frustrated, so I finally stopped hearing what you want to tell us. I really do want to hear what you have to say, but you seem to say so much that I just cannot keep up with it." This also should be followed by checking with others in the group to see if the feelings are shared or are peculiar to the leader. Even if they are peculiar to the leader, they warrant examination by Jones and the leader.

4. *Confrontation—Individual:* Jones—could you please shut up for a few minutes? We just aren't getting anywhere, and I really think it would be helpful if you'd be quiet and let a few other people have the floor." This kind of direct confrontation must be carried out in a generally supportive way. A mean or harsh statement may only press everyone into silence and thus not accomplish anything beneficial.

5. *Confrontation—Group:* "I think you should stop talking for a moment; I have something important to ask the others in this group. I've observed that Jones talks a great deal in this group; in fact, so much that none of the rest of you have any opportunity to participate. What I was wondering, however, is why you all have permitted Jones to monopolize the discussion?" This focus on the group's responsibility could also be coupled with an interpretation: "It may be that you all do not want to take any responsibility for working in this group and so eagerly permit Jones to monopolize the discussion."

This last possibility is an important one, especially when we retain our system's perspective on group process. In this view, we must recognize that the other group members may be supporting the domination by one member in order to avoid accepting their own responsibility for their group. The monopolizer, therefore, gets away with the domination but only because other members permit or even want it to be that way. By confronting the group with its behavior, the leader tries to focus on the total field within which the behavior occurs rather than locating the "blame" or full responsibility on the shoulders of the dominating individual.

Evaluation

Almost every intervention presented here is in the form of an open invitation for the individual or for the group to further explore and examine their behavior and its effects. If the invitation is not taken up by the individual or the members, then the leader must reevaluate the intervention approach. The leader may decide, for example, to probe the issue further, to offer additional interpretations or analyses, or perhaps to offer advice regarding a way of improving the equality of participation. A longer-term evaluation depends upon the extent to which the monopolizer stops monopolizing and the other group members take on more responsibility for handling their own participation.

DEALING WITH SILENCE AND APATHY

Issue

If one extreme of member participation involves the monopolizer, the other side involves the silent or apathetic member. The issue, here, however, is more complex. Silence and apathy may describe the behavior of the entire group. In either case, apathy and nonparticipation are some of the most typical and usually frustrating issues for a group's leader.

A few silent members may seem reasonable to the typical leader; yet one of the goals of leadership is to involve all members in the group. This calls for creating a climate within which the silent member feels secure enough to participate. A silent or apathetic group, on the other hand, rarely seems reasonable to any leader; it places the entire burden of responsibility and action on the shoulders of the leader and is not a desirable state of affairs. The leader's goal, therefore, is to understand the basis for several members' or the group's silence and low level of participation and then to intervene in ways designed to increase member involvement. Leaders who carry on soliloquies soon discover that not only are they doing all the work, but the important decisions are not carried out by the very persons who are expected to do this. An involved and actively participating membership is therefore an important goal to achieve.

Silence and apathy of either an individual or the group as a whole can have several different meanings. It is important for the leader to be sensitive to the range of meanings that are possible. Let us begin with an obvious but often ignored possibility. Silence and low participation for the group as a whole may be a direct result of the leader's own style of leadership. That is, silence may be a membership stype of response to an autocratic leadership style. The classroom teacher, for example, who always lectures and dominates the entire class, should not be so puzzled when no one responds to the request, "Are there any questions?" Similarly, leaders who make most decisions for their group in a unilateral manner, who dominate the discussion, who cut off members from particpating, and in other ways suggest that this is their group—that they are in charge, and that no one else counts as much as they do—should not be surprised to find member apathy and silence as the typical response. Thus, one of the first things to be examined when a leader encounters general groupwide apathy, nonparticipation, and silence is the leader's own style of leadership.

But silence also conveys other meanings as well. Borrowing from the discussion of Bradford, Stock, and Horwitz (1961), we can outline several reasons for general group silence and apathy:

1. The task facing the group does not seem important to members, even though it may seem important to the leader or to someone external to the group. For example, a health team may be confronted by an outside agency with an issue that members personally do not feel is particularly relevant. Their silence and general apathy reflects their attitude toward this particular task. Likewise, the leader may impose a task that he or she feels is critical to the group, but fails to inform or persuade others of its critical nature; thus general apathy reflects disinterest in what appears to be an irrelevent task. We are reminded here of a group of medical residents in Family Practice who were discussing various cases; the leader felt that the important task before this group was not simply to discuss a given case, but to examine the implications of members' disagreements concerning the case for their relationships to one another in the group. Members, however, did not see this interpersonal issue as relevant and so resisted the leader's efforts to get them to focus on this issue. Their resistance in this instance took the form of long silences and general disinterest in the entire discussion.

2. The group may feel frustrated if the task or issue seems beyond their present capabilities to handle. In this case, silence and apathy reflect the group's general frustration over its inadequacy to solve a particular problem.

3. Members sense that the issues they must face are frightening or threatening to the group as a whole or to a significant number of them, and so silence becomes a way of avoiding the threatening tasks. To return to the medical residents, it may have been that their silence was a result of their fear of examining their interpersonal relationships. That is, they did not simply define such a discussion as trivial and irrelevant to their major purposes but sensed that to engage in an examination of their own relationships would be too threatening and fearful; their silence and general nonresponsiveness reflected their avoidance of the threat. Recall Bion's concept of *flight* from Chapter 5; flight from a potentially controversial or frightening issue often takes the form of withdrawal into silence and apathy.

4. Silence and apathy, however, are also vehicles that convey the meaning of fight, conflict, and anger. A group may become silent and nonres-

ponsive as a way of dealing with its angry feelings or its internal conflicts. For example, a group may be dominated by a few argumentative members. Other group members may shy away from this form of participation; their silence reflects their inability to deal with the conflict, their fear of getting caught in the battle, or their anger over the dominance and fighting. In other cases, anger toward the leader may take the form of a withdrawal into silence. Much like the pouting child, a group or individual may likewise withhold participation as a way of expressing anger.

Most of the meanings of silence and apathy for the group as a whole can be applied to individual members as well. Thus extremely silent members may be frightened of the topic; may be angry at the leader, the group, or some of its members; may feel that the entire task before then is irrelevant and not properly suited to their purposes; and so forth. Needless to say, silence and apathy are important symptoms of underlying issues facing the individual or the group. It is important for the leader to work toward a diagnosis and intervention before the underlying problems destroy the effectiveness of the group or the contribution of the nonparticipating member(s).

Observation

On the face of it, silence and apathy would appear to be readily observable. Look around the room and spot persons whose participation seems low: they speak infrequently or not at all; they speak only when a direct question is asked of them; they do not respond when a general request for questions is made. There are many further manifestations of silence and apathy that can be observed. These include the following symptoms:

1. People appear to be bored or disinterested; they yawn, look around the room frequently, seem engaged in other activities than the task at hand, even doze or daydream.
2. The discussion seems to ramble on; members are unable to keep track of what they are talking about or why.
3. Few members actively contribute to the group's discussion or work; the burden falls on a few shoulders.
4. Members arrive late to meetings or absences seem unusually high; members leave early or excuse themselves frequently to leave for other more pressing matters.
5. Members seem more eager to set the time for the session to end

than to to deal with the present session itself; there is frequent checking of the time and watches; there is a high level of responsiveness and alertness only when the issues of closing the meeting comes up.

Diagnosis

We have already indicated several meanings that silence and apathy convey. The task of the leader is to make a careful assessment of the specific circumstances at hand in order to sharpen the diagnosis that is made. As we have suggested, apathy and silence can be a reflection of three related matters: leadership style, task issues, and interpersonal issues. Each of these provides a helpful clue to guide the leader's diagnostic search. For example, the leader must first carefully examine his or her own leadership style before jumping to other conclusions regarding the meaning of silence. This means that leaders must be able to process their own behavior (see Chapter 11). Although this is by no means an easy task, it is essential that leaders recognize that they are participants in the group as well as leaders; they can be significant determinants of whatever behavioral effects are observed. It should be obvious that a diagnosis that suggests that the silence and apathy are in response to the leader's style would require an intervention directed toward oneself.

The immediate circumstances surrounding the occurrence of silence provides additional material on which to base the diagnosis regarding its meaning. For example, if the group members have been generally responsive and generally equal in their participation but then suddenly become silent and withdrawn, leaders must ask themselves about the topic or issue that immediately preceded the silence. The discovery may be something as simple as noting, for example, that a conflict between two prominent members of the group has been uncovered; silence may reflect a fearful withdrawal from tampering with this conflict.

To take another example, the leader may have made an intervention that was followed by a silence. In checking out the intervention, the leader may note (as in an earlier example) that members were pushed into a topic or discussion that they felt was either irrelevant or too threatening to pursue. In either case, silence was their response.

Silence, especially of an individual member, does not always reflect a response to something in the immediately present setting; it may reflect some past wound within the group's or individual's life in general.

For example, in a group's early meetings, one member may have expressed her views quite openly and forcefully. If the group's response to this member was derisive laughter followed by some rather strong and angry rejections ("That's a stupid thing to say; I thought you knew better than that. Where did you get your training?") the member may become silent in subsequent sessions. Having been wounded once in the group, she fears to move out publicly to express herself again.

Members' past experiences are also reflected in their ongoing group behavior. An individual who is relatively insecure and not confident about himself or his views may be generally silent in group settings. Nothing specific has happened in this group to motivate this behavior; rather the silence reveals something external to the group that leads this person to be a minimal participant.

Interventions

As we have suggested throughout this discussion, the type of intervention that is attempted will depend on the nature of the diagnosis that is made. If leaders suspect that their own style of leadership is the major contributor to members' silence and apathy, then they not only must intervene to change themselves—they also must intervene by helping the group to work through and change its relationships with them. Specifically, leaders will have to check out their analysis against group members' own impressions: e.g., "I've noticed that there is a generally low rate of participation and involvement in this group. I was wondering if you are responding to the way I'm doing things. Is that contributing to your silence and apathy?"

Unfortunately, there is no magic in handling interpersonal relations; thus a leader who has dominated the group and led autocratically and then suddenly appears to be changing stripes may receive a non-commital, silent response to a question about leadership style. However, leaders who diagnose their own style as a major contributor to the group's silence must both work actively to change that style and also bring this possibility to the attention of the group. Intervention must be made at two separate but related points: the leader's own behavior and at the group level. The former involves leaders' effort to change their own behavior; the latter involves inviting the group members to respond to the leadership style (e.g., "How is my mode of leadership affecting this group?") and to help negotiate a different style, one that is more conducive to the members' involvement and participation.

Other interventions follow from the diagnosis of the meaning of silence and apathy. For example, the leader may suspect that the group is apathetic because the members think the task before them is not relevant or important. The leader can intervene by suggesting: "I've noticed that there is a general boredom with today's discussion. I wonder if people here feel that what we are doing is not really relevant?" This must be followed up with additional efforts to explore members' feelings about what they are doing and what they would like to be doing: "How do you feel about today's group? Are there things that you would prefer us to be doing or talking about?"

If leaders sense that the problem facing the group is members' feelings of inadequacy regarding their task, they can intervene by confronting that possibility: "I sense that people don't feel up to handling the issue we are dealing with. Is this generally the way people here feel?" Or leaders may sense that the group's inadequacy stems from lack of structure and organization; they can then intervene to facilitate the development of that structure: "I think that we've all been fumbling about for some time now, not really sure of what to do or how to go about dealing with the problem we're facing. I think it may be helpful if we can develop an agenda of important issues that we must deal with. That is, it may be helpful if we break the larger problem down into smaller parts and tackle each part one at a time. We may find this less frustrating."

If the diagnosis is of silence based on an interpersonal issue, such as fear, anger, or some related emotion, then the leader must decide either to intervene by offering an interpretation ("I wonder if people here are angry at what I've done?" "I wonder if we are afraid to bring up that topic because it may bring bad feelings out into the open") or decide not to intervene, but simply to let the silence pass. This latter approach has much merit, especially when the group has otherwise been moving along well and functioning effectively together. In this case it might take the group too far afield to begin to probe the underlying meanings and bases of the silence when it may just be a passing matter that is better left untouched, given the other purposes and agenda items of the group.

In many groups, an individual's silence should be left alone and untouched; the purpose of the group may not be best served by an attempt to make the group comfortable for a member if such an effort would require the use of too much group time and energy. In the end, it becomes a matter for careful judgment. Leaders must assess the meanings of silence and apathy and the general purposes of the group; they must then judge whether those purposes can be served by declining to intervene in any particular case. Silence, especially of one or a few individuals or as a passing matter within a group, may sometimes be handled best by nonintervention.

Continued silence and apathy, however, are another matter; these must be dealt with actively by the leader.

Evaluation

A successful intervention should be followed by the group's or an individual's overcoming the silence, working through the issue that motivated it, and continuing to function again. One of the best outcomes possible, of course, is that group members become better able to monitor their own behavior and facilitate their own process. In this case, members help one another break free from their silence; members take on increasing responsibility for their own actions and the success or failure of their group; members begin to examine, evaluate, and intervene in their own process—they begin to make their own interpretations of their silences and shorten what otherwise could be a lengthy and time-consuming process. For example, members may realize that when they are silent it means they may be shying away from an important issue that is threating; thus, they quickly try to identify that issue so that they can work more directly and immediately to restore full participation and involvement in their group. Successful interventions, therefore, do not only deal with the short-term issue of silence and apathy but also lay the groundwork for the group to use its own resources to deal with apathy or silence whenever it appears.

DEALING WITH EMOTIONAL OUTBURSTS

Issue

It is the rare group that is formed with the specific task or purpose of encouraging emotional outbursts such as anger and crying. Most groups with which the health professional is involved tend to have cooler norms: members adopt a view that is not hospitable to any excessive display of emotions. Even groups that are formed with the purpose of exploring members' personal experiences and feelings tend to be fearful of any real emotional display. Talking about emotions and feelings may be approved; "doing" the emotions, however, tends to be something of which most disapprove. That group norms tend to forbid or disapprove of actual emotional displays, however, does not mean that emotional outbursts will be absent. Feelings can and often do run high. Anger between members may suddenly break out; or a member may be touched by something that is taking place and begin to cry.

Given the high probability that most groups do not approve of emotional outbursts, the likely response when one occurs is silence, withdrawal, and avoidance. The leader then faces a member who has suddenly let loose a strong feeling and a group that fails to deal with it except by denying its existence. The task for the leader is to intervene helpfully for both.

There are really two related issues. The first involves helping the individual deal with the feelings that have been expressed and with the likely embarassment over having lost control in a setting that may be inhospitable and nonsupportive. The second involves helping the group develop a more responsible and less avoiding attitude toward such occurrences as well as to explore, where appropriate, the meaning and implication of the outburst in relation to the group's own functioning. This latter point can be especially important for the leader to work with.

In many instances, it is useful to think of the emotionally expressive member as a barometer of the entire group's climate. That person's outburst may be indicative of some underlying tensions within the group as a whole. The individual has lost control and openly expressed what many others might be feeling and experiencing. If this is the case, then the leader must make a special effort to relate the member's outburst to more generally shared group issues. The outburst can thereby become a valuable and important learning experience for the entire group. It is not simply that one member for some mysterious reason has lost control; rather, one member (perhaps with less control than others, a lower boiling point) has openly given vent to feelings that others may also be experiencing.

The two most common emotional displays in groups involve anger and crying. An open display of sexual feelings (e.g., kissing), while a possibility that would likewise have to be dealt with, seems less typical than the other two expressions. We will concentrate our discussion, therefore, around anger and crying. The techniques, however, are applicable whatever form the particular outburst may take.

Observations

Anger can be a very subtle as well as a very direct pattern of behaviors. A true outburst of anger is not difficult to observe: a loud, shouting voice, flushed face, tremors, body postures indicative of fighting. Fists may be clenched; short, choppy movements may be made; speech may be disjointed with a rapid rush of words. Cooler forms of the angry outburst may involve a person who is bordering on a complete loss of control and so seems intent on self-containment: the person may become rigid, leaning forward as though to lunge, yet getting white hands from holding on so tightly to retain control.

In similar manner, crying can range from a readily observed outburst of tears to a more subtle form. In the latter case, one can usually observe tears welling up in the person's eyes; the head is cast downward; they may wring their hands; their lips may tremble; they may withdraw or try to—e.g., cover the face, turn away from the group.

Diagnosis

The diagnostic issue involves an attempt to understand the basis for the member's outburst and also to locate similar feelings within other members of the group. The angry outburst, for example, can represent extreme frustration with what is going on in the group. It can also represent intense disagreement and conflict between members. For some, an angry outburst could represent a way of grabbing for attention. It also often represents "the last straw," reflecting a buildup of unexpressed feelings that finally reach a breaking point. In this instance, the precipitating event may be relatively minor; we must probe into past events in order to understand the intensity of the present response.

Anger, of course, generates anger. Thus, an outburst from one member may be the end point of an escalating cycle that has been building up within the group: i.e., Fred is humorously sarcastic to Bob, who replies with an intense angry comment to Fred who responds with a still more intense jibe at Bob, who finally breaks loose with an angry tirade that embarasses and silences everyone.

Crying can occur when one member hears something within the discussion that taps some deep-lying feeling within them: e.g., a nurse whose father has recently died suddenly bursts into tears when the group begins to discuss a patient's death. Crying can also represent anger. This may seem paradoxical, but some who consider that the open expression of anger may be inappropriate begin to cry when they are furious. Crying also occurs when people are so overwhelmed by what they are experiencing that they have no behavioral options other than to cry.

Crying when one is happy is another well-known possibility. Some psychoanalytically oriented theorists (e.g., Weiss, 1952; 1971) have suggested that people cry finally when they feel secure enough to let those feelings emerge into their consciousness. This kind of "crying at the happy ending" suggests that only when we have been reassured that the ending is happy can we permit ourselves to have the sad and tender feelings that we otherwise blocked out. Thus, we may diagnose some crying as indicative of the person's having reached a point of greater security with the group; they finally feel comfortable enough to let themselves cry.

Given the wide range of meanings that can be represented by anger or crying, one of the first tasks facing the leader is to determine what the outburst represents for the member. The intervention strategies, therefore, must include ways to further explore the meanings of such outbursts even while helping support the individual member and helping the group examine the relevance of the outburst to their own functioning.

Interventions

Diagnostic interventions are designed to help the leader and others gain a better sense of the meaning of an outburst; *supportive interventions* are designed to help the member, who may feel embarrassed by the behavior, to deal with the follow-up residues of their outburst. *Group-centered interventions* are designed to help the group members explore both their feelings about what has occurred and the degree to which they too share some of the member's feelings and experiences (i.e., the more general implications of the outburst for the group as a whole).

To help clarify the meaning of the outburst, the leader has several intervention possibilities. The leader may immediately reflect the feelings: "You sound (look) very angry." The leader may provide support in order to help the member clarify the meaning of their outburst: "You must really be upset; let's talk about it." Support and clarification may take the form of saying, for example, "I want you to know that I see your pain and I would like to help." The leader would then pause, using this intervention as an invitation for the member to continue.

If the nature of the outburst has been extreme—for example, anger that is more than verbal, in fact is overtly physical, or crying that is heading into an hysterical loss of control—one of the first tasks facing the leader is to restore some degree of control. This often requires some actual physical intervention: e.g., getting up and restraining the angry person or embracing the crying person. These are also supportive gestures; they help the person regain some of the lost control, so that they can join in the process of clarification.

Diagnostic interventions can also follow from the leader's interpretations and analyses of the likely meaning of the emotional outburst. These would take the form of testing the leader's analyses rather than being declarations of fact: "You began to cry when we started talking about death. Has there been a recent loss in your own life?" "Your anger at Marge seems out of proportion to what she actually said to you; I wonder if it's got something to do with your attitude toward women?"

It is important for the leader to be supportive while seeking to gain clarification. Likewise, it is important for the leader to invite and encourage the member to examine what has taken place; the leader should avoid pushing, leaving no way out but further retreat into emotional display: "Is this something that you can talk about now?" If the member indicates that he would prefer to wait a while (until some composure is regained), it is then important for the leader to open the invitation again later. That is, the leader should check back with the member and not abandon him after having invited him to examine the situation. This will also help the group members develop increased trust in one another and the ability to be secure in their expressions.

Assuming that the leader has been able to provide support and encouragement for the member and helped her clarify for herself and others the bases of the outburst, it is important for the leader to bring the experience back to the group-centered focus. Recall that the individual member's outburst may reflect sensitivity to an issue that is more generally shared. To test this out the leader can ask the group members directly to get in touch with their own feelings and to share them within the group:

A group of parents of handicapped children is discussing the difficulties they are experiencing, when suddenly one member begins to cry. The leader helps support that member while encouraging her to explore her crying. The member speaks about her feelings of personal guilt and responsibility for having caused her child's handicap. The leader suspects that this one member's feelings are not unique but are more general to the entire group. Thus, the leader invites the other parents to explore their own feelings, asking, "How do some of the rest of you feel about this?"

By inviting the group members to explore their own feelings, the leader facilitates the involvement of others who may have wished to do this; the leader also helps reduce the distance and separation between the group as a whole and the particular member who had the emotional outburst; all of this, in turn, can help increase the sense of cohesiveness within the group, as members share experiences they might not otherwise have been able to share.

Evaluation

The evaluative issue involves the degree to which the leader's interventions have successfully managed the outburst. In the context we have been discussing, successful management involves at least three related issues: supporting the members who have engaged in the outburst; clarifying the meaning of the outburst; helping the group to examine its own feelings about the outburst and the issues that it represents to members of the group. Successful interventions will be reflected in any or all of the following ways:

—Increased sense of cohesiveness within the group
—Greater openness and willingness to share and talk about feelings
—Integration of the member into the group rather than his or her separation or complete withdrawal
—Ability of the group to face up to difficult matters as they occur rather than to shelve them until they arise later, perhaps with excessive intensity.

Successful interventions, rather than increasing emotional outbursts within a group, should in the long run actually decrease their occurrence. Many outbursts are excessive and disruptive because they occur after a lengthy buildup of tension that is not dealt with when it occurs (this is especially true of anger and frustration). As the leader creates a climate within which members can more openly examine their feelings, the leader will facilitate the development of mechanisms within the group that make future outbursts less likely and less disruptive.

DEALING WITH CONFLICT WITHIN THE GROUP

Issue

As a careful reading of the theories of group development suggests (Chapter 8), conflict is a normal stage in the life of most groups. It is not something, therefore, that by its very nature is bad or destructive; in fact, conflict is often indicative of liveliness and innovation in problem solving. This being the case, leaders should not uncritically set about to eliminate all conflict that arises within their group; the task, rather, should be to encourage the kind of conflict that can help the group to grow. The constructive use of conflict can become a vital resource to a group.

Having said that, we must also recognize that, carried to an extreme, conflict in the form of bickering, disagreements, nastiness, a tense atmosphere, and such can be more of a hindrance than a helpful resource for a group. It is important to be able to achieve the delicate balance between those conflicts that lead a group astray or into more difficulty and those conflicts that facilitate growth and innovative problem solving. The task for the leader is to be able to separate destructive conflict from its more constructive form and to help create a climate within which disagreements are dealt with in a reasonable and constructive manner.

There are some useful ways to evaluate whether a conflict is more destructive than helpful (from Bradford, Stock & Horwitz, 1961):

1. When a group is faced with what appears to be an impossible task, members' frustration over their inability to handle it may erupt in conflict within the group. Such conflict is more an expression of frustration and tension than of the kinds of substantive disagreements that are constructive. It is important for the leader, therefore, to evaluate whether the basis for the conflict within the group is frustration and tension rather than actual disagreements over policies, values, solutions, priorities, and so forth.

2. It is not unusual for members of many groups to be primarily concerned with their personal, individual tasks, especially those involving their own rank and status within the group or within the larger organization in which the group is located. In such cases, members may engage in disagreements and fights as vehicles for expressing or gaining status. Power struggles between individuals, each of whom is attempting to gain the center stage for themselves, or members who talk

mainly as a way of being heard by their superiors, typically produce conflicts within a group that are less than constructive.

3. Members may argue and disagree within the group as a reflection of their competing loyalties to outside groups. That is, the group may be composed of individuals who represent different outside groups. The issues that are raised within the group and the conflicts that occur thereby reflect these competing outside loyalties. These conflicts can often prove constructive, especially when the leader can help members relate their inside behavior to these external interests and loyalties and guide them toward some compromise functioning within the group.

4. Conflicts often arise within groups among persons who are all highly invested in the group and its work and who genuinely disagree about procedures, priorities, policies, interpretations, and so forth. These are the kinds of conflicts that can usually prove to be constructive rather than destructive. There are numerous reasons for members to have conflicts with others; when these conflicts are based on highly committed members' genuine differences in point of view and values, then the group can build upon these differences to develop unique, innovative solutions to problems and issues.

Observations

Bradford, Stock, and Horwitz (1961) provide us with some useful symptoms of the various types of conflict that are common within groups. In our previous listing, two bases of conflict were relatively nonproductive (frustration over the task and individual status and power expressions), whereas two other bases were potentially productive (outside loyalties and genuine differences in perspectives and values). The leader who would hope to make a preliminary diagnosis that differentiates between the nonproductive and the productive types will find the following observations helpful:

Some indications that the conflict is *nonproductively* based:

—Every time a suggestion is put forth, it is rejected as being too impractical or impossible.

—Members seem never to have enough time for the group and its tasks and get angry and impatient with one another.

—Members have little sense of what their group is all about, why it exists, what its functions are, and so forth; they are always confused and puzzled.

—Every time an idea is expressed, it is attacked and put down even before it gets fully developed or examined.

—Members line up quickly on one side or another and refuse to negotiate or compromise.

—Members engage in direct or subtle personal attacks on one another.

—The same issues and problems are continually repeated; no solutions are ever found or accepted.

—Members act in ways to win their point or avoid losing their point, showing little concern for or recognition of others or of the group.

—Much talk is self-centered; members seem to participate only when they can be at the center of the group's focus.

Some indications that the conflict is potentially *productive:*

—Members have a goal in mind that they generally agree on and are working toward.

—Members' comments are directed toward the task at hand.

—Members are generally receptive to listening to and hearing others, even though they may respond with disagreement and alternative points of view.

—Members encourage one another to participate, even those with differing points of view.

—Solutions to problems and issues are reached by rational discussion and compromise, and when reached tend not to recur again and again.

—The basis for members' disagreements are openly examined and critically evaluated.

The leader's observations of conflict must attempt to locate both the who and the what of the conflict. The leader must be sensitive to the participants who are involved and what the basis of their conflict is. The particular intervention strategy that is chosen will depend on the diagnosis that is made.

Diagnosis

As we noted, conflict can be built on a potentially productive or a potentially nonproductive base. In the former, the leader uses his or her observations to infer beneficial conflict and intervenes in ways to help the group negotiate these conflicts. In the latter, when the leader infers destructive conflict, working through may not be as useful as some more avoiding approach. There is some indication, for example, that when conflicts are potentially destructive, they should be avoided or played down rather than directly confronted. It becomes a matter for careful judgment and testing out, however.

The leader may sense, for example, that the basis of a conflict between two members involves each member's grab for power and status within the group. The leader recognizes this to be a nonproductive basis for conflict for the group as a whole; the decision is to ignore it and to direct the group away from getting caught up in such a personal struggle. On the other hand, the leader may judge it to be more beneficial for the group to face this issue directly; the decision is to intervene and call the group's attention to what appears to be taking place: "I feel that Smith and Jones are each trying to gain some points in this discussion, and I don't think this is helping us deal with the particular case we are working on. I wonder if you two could either cool it for awhile or let us all explore your behavior with you."

Interventions

Whatever intervention strategy the leader may employ, it is wise to intervene early rather than late. The earlier leaders are able to determine that conflict is present, the earlier they can intervene in the process; early intervention helps thwart an escalating cycle of unproductive conflict. In addition, early intervention that effectively negotiates a resolution to the conflict helps build a firm foundation for using constructive conflicts as a group resource. The group that sees that conflict can occur without tearing the group apart or taking the group too far from its immediate tasks will learn to voice and use conflict and disagreement rather than to shy fearfully away from any open expression of differences.

As with most leader interventions, those involving conflict are also most effective if they occur within a climate of cohesion and trust. A group of individuals who care little for one another or for their group as a whole, who have little trust in anyone including the leader, is not likely to be responsive to most types of conflict-handling interventions. Under such circumstances, the leader will first have to work to facilitate a trusting and cohesive climate within the group; only then can interventions be helpful. Within this general context, however, we can examine several kinds of intervention strategies that the leader can employ:

Interpretation:

I believe that we are having trouble making a decision in our group because we have some rather definite conflicts between various members. I think that we had better look at those conflicts before we try to do any other kinds of work here.

Reflect Behavior:

I've noticed that several members have been silent for quite some time now, that several others are talking a great deal but usually at cross-purposes, that we seem generally unable to keep ourselves focused on anything but fighting and disagreeing.

Reflect Feeling:

I'm not sure how the rest of you feel, but I'm getting annoyed and frustrated over the constant disagreement and bickering that is taking place. I think we have a job to do, and I'd like to get on with it.

Confrontation:

Ms. Carlton, I think you are angry with your supervisor because you feel that if this procedure is accepted, you will no longer have the kind of access to her that you previously had. You seem to feel that the procedure will distance you too much from your supervisor and put too much burden on you. Is that why you are so impatient and are acting so upset with the rest of us?

Voicing the Unmentionable:

I think that you are afraid of losing some power on your service and that is why you are acting so angrily in here, disagreeing with almost everything that is said, even before you give it a full hearing.

We have mentioned only several possible interventions; each is oriented toward pointing out to the individual and to the group that some kind of conflict is present and is thwarting their effectiveness in working together. As we noted earlier, however, our goal may involve helping a group to avoid facing its conflicts altogether.

Assuming that the goal is to help a group effectively use its conflicts, then the leader's task is not simply to point out that there are disagreements, but to help focus the group on these and on their basis; the next step is to facilitate the negotiation of a compromise. This task can be outlined in three separate steps:

—Support and legitimate disagreement and conflict

—Help clarify the basis and meaning of the conflict
—Help negotiate a compromise.

The intial step may involve something as simple as *supporting the idea and the legitimacy of conflict*: "I think we have several disagreements that are being expressed here and I for one think that's a sign of a healthy group." Supporting disagreement is often necessary: it helps members see that they can disagree and not lose their integrity as individuals; that they can disagree and not have their group dissolve; that disagreement can be a useful resource for their group.

Clarifying the basis of conflict, the second step, requires that the leader helps members focus on the actual basis of their disagreements with one another: "I know that the two of you are arguing, but I'm not sure if I fully understand what you are disagreeing about. Maybe you could each stop for a moment and just indicate what your position is." To take another example, the leader might intervene to provide his or her own clarification: "Mr. Zimmer, did you mean that you disagree with Ms. Alison because you feel that the interests of the family as a group are more important than the interests of the patient as an individual? If that is what you meant, then it seems that you and Ms. Alison disagree over the values that medical practice should attempt to implement. I think this is an issue that many of us may have opinions on and should discuss further."

The third step, *negotiating a compromise*, though by no means an easy matter, requires that the leader first focus members on the substantive bases for conflict. The leader and the members are then in a position to examine solutions that all parties can accept and that build upon those areas in which they overlap in their position. The interventions are designed to help members see what they share in common before they get lost in emphasizing ways in which they differ. Once their commonalities are expressed and examined, it becomes possible to see what avenues for satisfactory compromise between opposing perspectives are possible: "I hear Mr. Zimmer saying that he needs more assistance with his department; and I hear Dr. Samuels saying that he is so overloaded at present that he is not able to give anyone any more time. I also note that you both agree that something has to be done. I wonder if it is possible for us to examine some ways for Dr. Samuels to help out Mr. Zimmer's department while receiving help for his own department's patient overload."

Evaluation

The signs of successful conflict resolution will be noted when

—The same old conflicts do not continually emerge over and over again; real solutions that have some durability are achieved
—Members do not fear to express disagreements or to explore their basis and seek some compromise
—Innovative solutions result
—Group cohesiveness and trust seem high even in the midst of much substantive disagreement
—The group does not remain rooted either to an overidealized "honeymoon" or a constant state of warfare; differences as well as similarities are recognized and openly accepted.

Effective handling of conflict results when group members are better able to tolerate and directly deal with their disagreements. Ineffective handling of conflict results either in members' fearing ever to disagree lest all hell break loose or failing to make any progress because they are so burdened by dissension with which they cannot deal. The successful intervention, therefore, will not eliminate conflict from the group but will help the group to use conflict as a productive resource.

DEALING WITH NORMATIVE DEVIANCE

Issue

As we noted in our discussion in Chapter 4, all groups develop norms for the behavior that is expected of members. Deviance can be said to occur when a member or several members violate these norms. The typical group response to deviance includes the application of sanctions (e.g., punishment and rejection) and efforts to restore the deviant to proper behavior within the group. Much time may be spent in these efforts to get the deviant member to shape up and fit the group's normative expectations. This is valuable time that usually could be spent in other endeavors. Thus, from the viewpoint of effectiveness, deviancy within a group can deflect the group from its other, often more important activities.

But more than the group may be affected by deviance. Deviant members tend to be less satisfied with their group experience; they may feel anxious and tense. Because they are less valued and even attacked by other members, their self-esteem suffers. Any benefits that group membership can have tend to be lost upon the deviant who is disenfranchised from group involvement. Deviant members are more likely to terminate their membership, to arrive late, attend poorly, and in other ways disrupt the group and their own participation in it. Finally, research has suggested that deviants tend to be prime candidates for becoming casualties or being harmed by the group (Yalom, 1975; Lieberman, Yalom & Miles, 1973). In other words, the leader's responsibility both to the group and to the individual warrants a serious consideration of the deviant member of the group. The tendency is for both the group as a functioning unit and the deviant as an individual to suffer from deviant behavior.

Deviancy develops as a function of two factors: the particular norms of the group and the degree to which a group is open to tolerating deviation from these norms. A deviant, for example, could be someone who wears his hair long in a group that has short hair-length norms and that is intolerant of any variation from its norms. That same person in a more tolerant group may be a deviant in that the norms still call for short hair, but his deviancy does not disrupt him or the group, and does not lead to his rejection from the group; its higher level of tolerance permits a wide latitude of behaviors and appearances.

Given these two factors, the leader's efforts can be directed toward the deviant member's behavior, toward the group's norms, or toward the group's level of tolerance. For example, the leader can try to help the deviant member fit in better with the group; can try to counsel him out of the present group and into a different group; can help support him in his deviance by giving him a greater feeling of acceptance and belongingness. However, the leader can also try to help the group change its norms; can help the group become more tolerant in its norms and sanctions for deviancy; can help the group overcome its need for this particular member to change behavior even while the group does not agree to modify its norms.

Notice that the leader's goals involve helping the group as well as the deviant individual. Notice further that the accomplishment of these goals does not demand the single solution of changing the deviant. Rather, there are several possibilities. Deviancy from group norms is not bad or evil; it has consequences for both group and individual, however, that warrant careful leader judgment and intervention.

Observations

The major observational tasks facing the leader involve both a determination of the group's norms and a determination of the intensity of the effect of normative deviation on the individual and on the group. Members who embody and exemplify a group's norms will tend to be highly valued and turned to frequently for their opinions. Those who deviate from the norms will tend to be rejected and devalued by group members. We know that norms can pertain to almost any aspect of behavior or appearance. However, groups typically develop norms regarding such issues as appropriate conversation, appropriate clothing and mannerisms, an appropriate level of emotional expression, the appropriate way of relating to authority and leaders, appropriate ways of dealing with client populations and task issues.

Although we cannot observe norms directly, they can be inferred from our observations of members' behavior and group reactions. Thus our initial task, the determination of a group's norms, can be based on observing group responses to members. Leaders can ask themselves such questions as

—Who receives negative feedback and what about them evokes this feedback? Negative feedback can involve a direct expression—"How dare you come in here looking like that! Don't you know the proper attire for a nurse?" It can also be much more subtle and indirect, ranging from the way the member is looked at (e.g., with eyes and face saying "How dare you . . ."), to silence, nonresponsiveness, and even nonrecognition of the other (e.g., ignoring the person who deviates as though by failing to notice them or to respond to them, they'll disappear). Indirect expressions of negative feedback can also be noted from the ways in which people fight one another or disagree with one another. Scapegoating often reflects the existence of norms from which a member is deviating.

—Who gets the attention? Attention-getting members can often be used as "observational informants" for determining group norms. What about the person brings them so much of the group's attention?

—Who is turned to for opinions and seems to be valued and respected by the group? Again, one can infer a group's norms by observing persons who are most highly esteemed and valued by the group: e.g., members who, when they speak, are listened to; who command attention; who are turned to for their opinions before the group is willing to continue with its discussion; whose favor and approval is frequently sought.

—How would I, as a leader, feel in this member's shoes in this group?

(This is the as-if approach introduced in Chapter 9.) Leaders can ask themselves about the kinds of behavior that they would feel uncomfortable with in this group and the kinds of behavior that they feel to be appropriate. In other words, leaders use themselves as a guideline to understanding the group's norms.

The second observational task facing the leader involves a determination of how consequential the deviancy is on the individual and on the group. Several observational strategies are useful in this determination:

—Is the group repeatedly focusing its attention on a particular member who seems unable to change in ways to satisfy members?

—Does the group spend an inordinate amount of time talking about Ms. X or about issues that are brought up by Ms. X?

—Does the group forever return to Ms. X, putting all other matters aside?

—Does the presence of Ms. X evoke anger or resentment? Does Ms. X seem to have withdrawn (even physically) and become isolated from others in the group?

—Does Ms. X show signs of tension and anxiety or general discomfort?

Basically, the effects of the deviancy must be determined by observing the amount of time spent by the group in focusing on a given member (too much or too little can indicate trouble with that member) and by the nature of the response of that member: e.g., withdrawal, anxiety, tension.

Diagnosis

The diagnostic task facing the leader involves determining the basis for the member's deviancy and the group's response to it and the importance of the deviancy to the member and the group. The former question focuses on the meaning of the deviancy: e.g., Does it reflect specific anger on the part of the member? Is it a symptom of some more general disturbance? Is it a matter of cultural differences among members of the group? Is it a reflection of the group's intolerance?

The latter question focuses on the degree to which the deviant behavior is disruptive to the individual or the group. A diagnosis, for example, that the real problem is a more general disturbance might motivate the leader to try (where feasible) to counsel the deviant member out of the group or to help the group avoid its incessant, time-consuming and unfruitful focus on the deviant member. A diagnosis of a relatively minor disruption, for example, might motivate the leader simply to leave things alone, letting the matter pass. A diagnosis that suggest that the real problem lies with the group's rigid and intolerant norms might motivate the leader to address the group rather than the deviant member.

Interventions

The particular interventions that a leader uses are a function of understanding the meaning of deviancy and a decision about the appropriate target for the intervention. Thus, the leader may make *deviant-centered interventions* or *group-centered inventions,* or both. The former focuses attention on the deviant member and on the meaning of the deviancy. The latter focuses attention on the group's response to the deviant, the norms the deviant is violating, the importance of those norms to the group, its degree of tolerance, and so forth.

Let us suppose that the leader decides initially at least to implement deviant-centered interventions. The leader can then work to clarify the basis for the member's deviancy: e.g., Does it reflect a persistent personal habit (e.g., nail biting)? Does it reflect rejection of the group? Does it reflect anger directed toward the group? Does it reflect ignorance or insensitivity to the group's norms? Does it reveal some personal psychological conflict or need (e.g., the person's low self-confidence motivates him or her to continually solicit positive feedback from others; this constant solicitation proves annoying to others who value confidence in members and disparage displays of what they see as weakness)? Does it reflect a different cultural or class pattern (e.g., members of a different social class or culture may behave in ways that are appropriate to their own group but which violate the norms of the typical middle-class American culture)?

It is important to realize that the type of intervention chosen will reflect the leader's understanding of the meaning of the deviance for the individual and the group. A few examples will help clarify this issue:

—If the deviance means that the member is angry with the group or with someone in the group, then interventions must be directed toward the anger rather than the deviant behavior as such: "I've noticed that you always respond to others in this group with what I feel to be anger or resentment. This response seems to run against the grain of this group—we all seem to have agreed not to openly express our anger to one another—and it also seems to be further alienating you from the group. I think it would be helpful if we could talk some about your angry feelings."

—If the deviance reflects ignorance or insensitivity to the group's norms, then interventions can be directed toward helping the member and the group clarify just what these normative expectations are: "I've noticed that some members are annoyed at others' behaviors, but I'm not sure that we understand why. Perhaps it would be useful for us to look at the kinds of expectations we have for one another."

—If the deviance reflects a different cultural or class pattern, then interventions can be directed toward helping the member and the group learn about these cultural differences: "I think we have a great opportunity here to learn more about ourselves by examining our reactions to Ms. Chin; it seems that some of our reactions stem from our cultural differences. It might be very useful for us to understand these differences."

In more general terms, the intervention goal will usually involve opening up the deviant's behavior to group and self-examination. This may be done by reflective techniques: "Your behavior seems somewhat different than that of others in this group; it also seems to be disturbing to some. Maybe we should talk more about it." Or the leader might reflect feelings that he or she is experiencing or suspects that others in the group are experiencing: "I've noticed that whenever you talk, I get somewhat edgy and annoyed at you, as though you say things that people are not supposed to say in this group; I've also noticed some others in the room getting edgy. I wonder if we are feeling anxious and bothered because you act somewhat differently from the rest of us."

The leader can use supportive intervention to the same ends: "I really like some of the things you say and do in here. I've noticed, however, that you behave differently from many other members of this group and that this difference seems to trouble some people."

The leader may choose, on the other hand, to focus more on the group than on the deviant. In this case, interventions will be designed to help the group attend to the deviant's behavior and to their responses and feelings about it: "I've noticed that Alice's appearance is not generally the same as that of other members in this group and that people here seem to be offended by this. I wonder if this is something that we should all examine further?" Or the leader may more simply ask, "How do the rest of you feel about the way Alice dresses?"

It is very difficult to focus on the deviant without further separating that person from the group. Insofar as her separation poses a real problem for her and for the group, it is incumbent upon the leader to attempt to reintegrate the deviant even while calling attention to her unique status: "I'm concerned that some of us are responding negatively to Alice, and I'm not sure that this is good either for her or for our group. I know that we have many other things to do, but I feel that we must take some time out now to deal with our reactions to Alice."

The implication is that whatever specific intervention is selected, *support* is fundamental to handling any normative deviation. Deviants are rarely in a comfortable position in the group, whatever the basis or meaning of their deviancy. They are already separated from others by virtue of their deviant actions; calling attention to their behavior only further separates them. All intervention goals must build upon a firm foundation of support for the deviant, even when it is necessary to counsel them out of the group, work to help them modify or change their behavior, help the group better understand their reactions to the deviant, and so on.

Evaluation

A successful handling of the deviant will prove beneficial both to the group and to the deviant member. The benefit to the deviant, however, may not be a transformation into a nondeviating member; rather, it may more likely involve a change in which the deviancy is no longer disruptive to the group (e.g., excessively time-consuming) and the deviant member no longer suffers the negative consequences of rejection and alienation from the group. It is against this dual standard that leaders must measure and evaluate their success. If the group cannot extricate itself from a continued fascination and involvement with the deviant or if the deviant shows increasing signs of tension and anxiety, then the leader might well consider acting to help extricate the deviant from the group rather than continue with a membership that is disturbing to all.

These are not easy decisions to make; the goals, however, are sufficiently clear; and the various techniques of intervention must be chosen wisely in the service of these goals.

GETTING A GROUP STARTED

Issue

Place yourself in the position of being in a group that has just formed. What are some of the questions you might have? This will provide a useful clue about some of the important issues that are involved whenever a group is getting started. Three major kinds of questions would appear relevant to consider: questions of *who, what,* and *how.* That is, Who is here? What are we to do? How shall we proceed?

Who is here? If the members of the group all know one another from past contacts and work together, this may not seem to be as an important an issue as it would be in a group in which few persons know one another. Yet even with people who have worked together before, a group that is formed with a purpose that is different from their usual contacts will need to have this question answered.

> A nurse was asked by her church group to lead a group dealing with children's sexuality. She was a regular member of the church, as were the parents with whom she was meeting to develop the program for their children. Although everyone in the room had had many previous contacts with one another, they had never before convened around the topic of sexuality. Thus, one of their opening issues involved such questions as: "Who are these other people?" "Can I trust them when I talk about sexual matters?" "Who is this nurse?"

The example suggests that the "who" question is concerned not only with the other members but also with a group's leader or organizer.

The "who" question also contains the issue of trust: Who in here can I trust? Who can I rely on? Who are my friends and allies? Who are my adversaries? As the example suggests, members may know "who" the others in their group are; after all, they have been together in the same church for many years. But they do not know much about "who" these people are in matters of sexuality (the group's purpose for being organized); they do not know whom they can trust to hear about their own views, to respect what they have to say, to listen with caring and concern for their own worries and issues.

Discovering the variety of meanings to the "Who" questions thus becomes an important matter in opening a group. It is rarely sufficient simply to begin without some efforts directed toward these issues. Introductions are an important first step. Other interventions will be examined shortly.

Other important questions also exist at the beginning: Why are we here? What are our goals and purposes? Members are generally not only concerned with who is there, but why they have all been convened—i.e., *what* their purposes are. It is imperative for the leader to realize that although he or she may know the reasons they have convened, the members may either not know this reason or may have other goals and purposes of their own. Thus, an early task in the life of a group must be to focus on goals and purposes—"what we are here to do."

How shall we proceed? Members may know who is there and what the joint purposes are, but need help in defining and clarifying how they shall go about accomplishing their goals. Especially if the leader hopes to facilitate a democratically functioning group, it will be important to begin early to develop this style and help members work within its framework.

Observations

There is much to be observed at the opening or first several meetings of the group. Anticipating that issues of who, what, and how will be salient to members provides the leader with an opportunity to focus on the content of what is being said and especially on what is being implied though not directly said. Early sessions in an ongoing group or in the first part of even a short-term group must be devoted to establishing rapport among members and between members and the leader; a sense of trust must emerge.

The absence of trust or anxiety over trust can appear in several forms. (1) Members may be reluctant to open up and talk directly to one another about what they are feeling or about their opinions. Little sharing takes place. (2) The leader may feel that he or she is the prod, doing much of the talking and much of the work. (3) There may be frequent indirect reference to issues of "trust" ("The hospital administration is simply not to be trusted") that may also be reflections of that same issue existing within the group. (4) Statements that are made may get little or no response from others. It is as though nonresponse is used for self-protection ("If I let you talk without probing and responding, then you'll let me talk uncritically and this makes life much safer"). (5) Topics may ramble without much direction, almost disconnected, as though persons are not yet ready to converse in anything more than a polite or superficial manner.

Frustration over a lack of clarity regarding the goals and purposes of the group (the "what" question) may also be readily observed: (1) Members may appear restless and bored; perhaps few will participate. (2) Direct as well as indirect expressions of confusion may frequently occur ("I'm not sure what I'm expected to say"; "I wish we could get some kind of structure to this session"). (3) Frustration may lead to impatience, irritability, and anger; thus, expressions of any of these may occur in response to a need for clarity over goals and purposes.

Finally, "how" issues may be revealed in several ways: (1) Members may not know how to relate to the leader; they may request (directly or typically indirectly), more leadership, more structure, more direction. (2) Members may not be sure how they should go about dealing with the task they face, what procedures should be used, who should speak, how decisions should be made, and so forth

Diagnosis

As we have noted, who, what and how questions are relevant to the early life of most groups. These will crop up in many direct as well as disguised forms; the leader should anticipate their occurrence and be prepared to diagnose group or individual difficulties in their terms. In recognition that groups have phases (see Chapter 8 for further details on group stages of development), the leader should know that orientation and inclusion issues (in the form of who, what, and how questions) predominate early in the life of a group. This provides the leader with a ready framework within which to diagnose many of the problems that are likely to occur early on. In other words, knowing the most likely questions and issues that exist when a group is just getting started will help the leader's diagnosis of the members' often unstated agenda items. Members may not directly confront any of these issues; however, they form a part of the unstated or hidden agenda which leaders can use to guide and inform their specific interventions.

Interventions

Because the three major initial issues involve who, what, and how, the leader's interventions must come directly to grips with each of these questions as they are revealed by members' interactions. In the beginning, the best tactic for the leader to follow is to anticipate these issues and lay the groundwork for handling them even before observing their presence. Rather than waiting to observe signs that the group is concerned with "who" (i.e., trust and inclusion), for example, the leader should direct efforts toward helping the group answer these unasked questions.

Early introduction of members, asking them to say something briefly about themselves is important. It is likewise important for leaders to introduce themselves and inform the group about who they are. Anticipating that "inclusion" issues are important, the leader from the beginning should invite members to join in and to participate: e.g., asking for introductions; inviting feedback and expressions of opinions and points of view.

Trust does not occur magically; it evolves from a context in which members begin to feel secure with one another and with their group leader. The leader can contribute significantly to this sense of security by acting in supportive and encouraging ways. Leaders who open with a fast-fire critique are clearly informing members that they are in a risky situation—beware. Expressions of support for members who begin to participate; inviting members to join in, to share, and to be heard: all of these are helpful early interventions that help establish a sense of rapport and trust. Modeling desirable behavior (e.g., supportive, attentive listening, concern) can likewise be most helpful in early leader interventions.

Questions of "what" (What are our goals and purposes?) must also be dealt with very early. In this too, the leader's ability to anticipate this issue can help short-circuit problems that might otherwise develop. Interventions here should help members focus on their own purposes for the group; likewise, purposes that the leader has or that are given to the group from "external sources" (e.g., hospital administration) must be openly introduced and examined. Much opening work must be devoted to an expression of goals and purposes (members, leaders, organizations), and to a negotiation over the goals and purposes and the priorities of the group.

The leader's interventions must help members develop their own goals, negotiate with others over what the group's goals will be, and set priorities. The latter offers a useful way of organizing what may appear to be diverse sets of goals by locating some of them at the top of the list for immediate consideration and action and others lower down for later consideration and action.

Interventions that are designed to deal with questions of "how" are also necessary for early work. Let us suppose that the leader desires to establish a democratic leadership style, one in which members adopt the following as their own procedures of operation: taking responsibility for their group; working together toward commonly defined goals; negotiating decisions rather than accepting the will of the most dominant member or leader. In this case the leader must intervene with this style from the very beginning.

It is often useful for the leader to inform the group about his or her preferred mode of leading: "I prefer to help facilitate group discussion rather than to lead in the typical manner; thus I see my role as helping members participate, to invite your participation and involvement in the group." It is likewise important for leaders to adopt this style in their mode of interacting in the group: e.g., to invite members' participation; to help clarify; to summarize, paraphrase, and reflect; to process the ongoing interaction. Creating a group in which a democratic style exists and in which members take responsibilities for processing and providing feedback to one another about what their group is doing—all this must start with the first session.

Evaluation

A successful beginning is one that deals with the three opening issues that confront all groups: Who is here? What are our goals and purposes? How shall we go about working together? Failure to handle the issue of "who" will lead to low trust and insufficient rapport for the group to work well together. Failure to handle the issue of "what" will lead to high levels of frustration and confusion, withdrawal into apathy, and reluctance to participate further in so ill-defined and disorganized a group. Failure to handle the "how" question will lead to inability to act—that is, an inability either to make decisions or to act upon and implement the decisions that are made. Success, on the other hand, exists when members begin to feel that they know who is there; they develop a sense of reasonable security in participating and in sharing their own views and opinions; they have a sense that they know their purposes and how the group can proceed to handle them and reach their negotiated goals; they feel that their own interests have been merged into the group's purposes and that their needs will be taken care of as the group goes about its business.

TERMINATING A GROUP

Issue

Terminating a group can involve several things: something as simple as the end of one meeting when many others are still planned; the end of a group that has been meeting together for sometime but is now ending; the end of a group that has convened only once or a few times. To end, though it carries a different intensity of feeling in each case, still poses certain issues with which the leader and members must deal. For example:

1. What have we accomplished in our time together?
2. Have our goals been achieved or have we failed?
3. How do we feel about leaving one another? Is there a sense of loss?
4. Is this really the end or just a break? Do we need to continue our group or arrange for additional times together?

Long-term groups or even short-term groups that have developed a strong, close bond face an especially difficult issue in terminating. Terminating in such instances implies *loss*; the usual response to loss is grieving and often anger. If a group has developed close relationship, then on terminating, people anticipate the loss of their group and relationships; even though some individuals may continue to have contact, the group as a living entity will be over. Members may need to grieve over this loss; one important component of that grieving is often a sense of anger: e.g., "You are all abandoning me."

Short-term groups in which no substantial personal bonding has occurred will tend to experience much less loss and less need to grieve; such a group will nevertheless have terminating issues typically involving more task-related matters and matters of personal self-esteem. If the interpersonal bonds have not been intense, then their termination will not be as critical an issue as in those groups in which such bonds have developed. However, task-related issues will be important. In particular, members' self-esteem may be embedded in their group success or failure on their task: "If we failed to reach our goals, am I responsible for that failure?" Thus, termination can mean "failure" or "success," lowered self-esteem or higher self-esteem.

Needless to say, the leader cannot simply come to the end of the life of a group and leave without helping the group deal with its termination issues. This means sufficient time must be allowed for the group to examine those issues (not the last 2 minutes of the final meeting) and to work through members' feelings about their group and its accomplishments. The leader can anticipate members' denial and avoidance of terminating issues; this means that the leader bears special responsibility to help the group probe the meaning of its termination. The leader, likewise, will have to be able to interpret symptoms of termination: e.g., lateness, apathy, refusal to engage in deep or meaningful discussions, angry, seemingly unfocused feelings, premature termination, and withdrawal. The latter is especially important in that many groups will try to terminate long before their actual end and thus withdraw all their involvement, leaving the last several sessions with no action, no decisions, no caring.

Observations

Knowing that terminating is an important issue, the leader must be prepared to observe early warning signs. As noted, these can include a diverse array of members' behaviors that are linked to terminating. (1) Members who formerly talked rather openly and easily together now may seem to have reverted to modes of defensiveness and superficiality. (2) Anger may seem to be prevalent as though members are upset with their leader or with one another, with no clear or apparent "stimulus" other than the imminent end of the group. (3) Conversation may shift toward discussions of death, dying, failure, loss, or some other such theme that suggests the feelings that termination bring to the forefront. (4) Members may begin to talk about or make plans for meeting beyond the final time; some urge a continuation of the group as if by continuing they can avoid dealing with their feelings of termination. (5) Some members may begin to withdraw, to come late to meetings, to miss meetings, to act as though the group is over and no longer a relevant matter for them.

Diagnosis

We diagnose that the issue is one of termination from a combination of behaviors we observe and our awareness that the time for the group's ending is near. Behavior early in the life of a group that is scheduled for ten meetings means something different from what appears to be that same behavior during the ninth meeting: e.g., talking about loss and grief early in a group may refer to some external issue, whereas that same talk during the ninth meeting may be indicative of concern with this group's own termination and the feelings that are then surfaced.

We have suggested two separable though related diagnoses on what we have termed termination issues: the one focuses on *interpersonal issues* and themes; the other centers on *task-related issues* and themes. Interpersonal issues are very likely whenever group members have established an intense bonding to one another or to the leader. These issues, involving loss, helplessness, vulnerability, grief, and anger, are also especially likely to occur among those members who have shared or disclosed more of themselves in the group. They can feel the loss most keenly or be most angry that "they gave," but there is no longer any time for others to reciprocate. Taking risks and disclosing oneself in a group not only helps cement bonds of trust and caring; it also lays a foundation for often intense feelings of loss on termination.

Task-related termination issues, as we have noted, are concerned especially with feelings of success and failure; basically these are matters of individual self-worth and self-esteem. Having been a member of a group that stated its goals and accomplished them can make termination a positive experience by comparison with a group that failed to reach its goals or produced a product or made decisions that few were pleased with. In the latter case, termination, although it may seem like a relief, can also contain the seeds for self-doubt and lowered self-esteem. Such possibilities are at least worthy of being explored within the group.

Interventions

The primary task of the group leader is to help the group engage its own termination issues, face them and work them through. This means that the leader must recognize the symptoms of termination and help the group interpret these: "I sense that several of you are very angry that we have only two meetings remaining. I've noticed that people seem to be coming in later and later. Perhaps we are concerned with our termination and should look at how we feel about this." Or the leader might observe that members seem unable to leave any given meeting; they hang around and wait and wait, not wanting to be the first to leave. This too might be interpreted to the group as a termination issue.

The leader's role is to intervene by interpreting behaviors as reflections of termination and by asking the members to probe their feelings about termination. This can often be facilitated by the leader's own sharing. How does he or she feel about this group coming to an end? Leaders' feelings often provide useful clues about members' feelings. If the leader genuinely feels a sense of loss, it is likely that other members will also share this feeling. If the leader feels frustrated and angry at the group for having failed to work well, it is likely that other members will share many of these same feelings. Thus, interventions can be helpfully guided by leaders' analysis of their own feelings on termination.

Knowing that termination themes involve loss as well as self-esteem will help determine the leader's interventions. The leader can directly ask members how they feel about their group's work together. Do they feel a sense of pride in what they have done or a sense of failure? Do they feel themselves responsible for what has taken place or not responsible?

Two critical issues that the leader faces involve either terminating too early or avoidance and denial of termination. In either case, the leader must intervene. The first situation requires interventions that remind members that they still have much time together and that any behavior that appears like termination is not appropriate this early. The latter calls for the leader to confront members with their worries about terminating, interpreting their behavior in these terms, and then help members openly explore and examine their feelings.

Evaluation

Successful termination will leave members with a valid sense of their experience and work together. They will come away not denying their involvement and self-disclosures nor being embarrassed or ashamed, but rather remembering the good times, the good feelings, the caring and concern that they and others shared. A good termination, in other words, will help members as they approach and enter other group experiences. A poor termination can sour members on interpersonal relations; they will come away feeling that they became involved but to no end, to no purpose other than the pain and anger of loss.

Successful termination, even when group members have not worked well together and have basically failed to accomplish the group tasks, will leave members with a knowledge of why they failed and how they can proceed better in their next group or committee involvement. In other words, successful termination will help members learn from their failures as well as enjoy their successes. Leaders must evaluate their own success in handling termination issues in these terms. Their goals will have been accomplished if failure becomes a building block for later success and if self-disclosure and intense bonding becomes a welcome rather than a frightening future prospect.

SUMMARY AND CONCLUSIONS

This chapter has sought to introduce the prospective group leader to some of the major questions that are asked and some of the ways of thinking about and providing answers to those questions. A general intervention model was introduced. This model calls on the leader to undertake a pre-intervention analysis, adopt an intervention strategy based on that analysis, and finally to evaluate the success of the intervention chosen. Pre-intervention questions require the leader to define the nature of the problem or issue. This includes examining why something is a problem, what observations are made, and what diagnosis emerges from an understanding of the nature of the problem and these observations. Intervention strategies vary as a function of the specific diagnosis made; they include the entire range of feedback and processing approaches we have considered in this and other chapters (e.g., Chapter 11). Post-intervention evaluation requires leaders to gauge the success or failure of their analysis and intervention in terms of certain criteria, examined in this chapter.

Whatever the particular intervention approach adopted, effective leadership must build upon four critical elements: genuine care and concern for the group, its members, and its functioning together; knowledge of group process concepts and theories; development of the perceptual and interpersonal skills needed to intervene in a group's ongoing process; sensitivity to oneself and one's impact on group process as a participant-observer. These four factors are like the legs of a table; any one that is missing causes wobbling, uncertainty, insecurity.

This text (and this chapter) has stressed three of these four elements; the fourth—genuine care and concern—while not as readily taught, often derives from the sense of self-confidence that the other three elements provide. As individuals develop a solid foundation in group process concepts and theory, the perceptual and interpersonal skills required to intervene in a group, and awareness of themselves as a participant in the process of the group, they can acquire a greater interest in and concern for the group they lead or in which they are members. It is difficult not to develop this genuine concern once we know something about how groups function and about the ways we can intervene to facilitate the improvement of that functioning.

References

Adams, J. S. Inequity in social exchange. In L. Berkowitz (Ed.), *Advances in experimental social psychology*. Vol. 2. New York: Academic, 1965.

Allport, G. W. & Odbert, H. S. Trait names: A psycholexical study. *Psychological Monographs*, 1936, *47*, Whole No. 211.

Argyle, M. & Dean, J. Eye contact, distance and affiliation. *Sociometry*, 1965, *28*, 289–304.

Argyris, C. Dangers in applying results from experimental social psychology. *American Psychologist*, 1975, *30*, 469–485.

Argyris, C. The incompleteness of social psychological theory. *American Psychologist*, 1969, *24*, 893–908.

Argyris, C. Theories of action that inhibit individual learning. *American Psychologist*, 1976, *31*, 638–654.

Argyris, C. & Schon, D. *Theory in practice*. San Francisco, Calif.: Jossey-Bass, 1974.

Asch, S. E. *Social psychology*, Englewood Cliffs, N.J.: Prentice-Hall, 1952.

Bales, R. F. Adaptive and integrative changes as sources of strain in social systems. In A. P. Hare, E. F. Borgatta, & R. F. Bales (eds.), *Small groups*. New York: Knopf, 1955.

Bales, R. F. The equilibrium problem in small groups. In A. P. Hare, E. F. Borgatta, & R. F. Bales (Eds.), *Small groups*. New York: Knopf, 1955.

Bales, R. F. *Interaction process analysis: A method for the study of small groups*. Cambridge, Mass.: Addison-Wesley, 1950a.

Bales, R. F. A set of categories for the analysis of small group interaction. *American Sociological Review*, 1950b, *15*, 257–263.

Bales, R. F. *Personality and interpersonal behavior*. New York: Holt, Rinehart & Winston, 1970.

Bales, R. F. Task roles and social roles in problem-solving groups. In E. E. Maccoby, T. M. Newcomb, & E. L. Hartley (Eds.), *Readings in social psychology* (3rd ed.). New York: Holt, Rinehart & Winston, 1958.

Balint, M. *The doctor, his patient, and the illness.* New York: International Universities Press, 1957.

Bass, B. M. *Leadership, psychology, and organizational behavior.* New York: Harper & Row, 1960.

Bateson, G., Jackson, D., Haley, J., & Weakland, J. Toward a theory of schizophrenia. *Behavioral science,* 1956, *1,* 251–264.

Bavelas, A. Communication patterns in task-oriented groups. *Journal of the Acoustical Society of America,* 1950, *22,* 725–730.

Benne, K. D., & Sheats, P. Functional roles of group members. *Journal of Social Issues,* 1948, Vol. IV.

Bennis, W. B. & Shepard, H. A. A theory of group development. *Human Relations,* 1956, *9,* 415–438.

Berger, P. L. & Luckman, T. *The social construction of reality.* New York: Doubleday, 1966.

Bernstein, B. *Class, codes, and control, I: Theoretical studies towards a sociology of language.* London: Routledge & Kegan Paul, 1971.

Bernstein, B. (Ed.). *Class, codes and control, II: Applied studies towards a sociology of language.* London: Routledge & Kegan Paul, 1973.

Bexton, W. H., Heron, W., & Scott, T. H. Effects of decreased variation in the sensory environment. *Canadian Journal of Psychology,* 1954, *8,* 70–76.

Biddle, B. J. & Thomas, E. J. (Eds.). *Role Theory: Concepts and Research.* New York: Wiley, 1966.

Bion, W. R. *Experiences in groups.* New York: Basic Books, 1959.

Birdwhistell, R. *Introduction to kinesics: An annotation system for analysis of body motion and gesture.* Louisville, Ky.: University of Louisville Press, 1952.

Blom, J. P. & Gumperz, J. J. Some social determinants of verbal behavior. In J. J. Gumperz and D. Hymes (Eds.). *Directions in sociolinguistics.* New York: Holt, Rinehart & Winston, 1972.

Blumer, H. Sociological implications of the thought of George Herbert Mead. *American Journal of Sociology,* 1966, *71,* 535–544.

Borgatta, E. F., Couch, A. S. & Bales, R. F. Some findings relevant to the great man theory of leadership. *American Sociological Review,* 1954, *19,* 755–759.

Bowlby, J. *Attachment and loss, Vol. 1. Attachment.* New York: Basic Books, 1969.

Bowlby, J. *Attachment and loss, Vol. 2. Separation.* New York: Basic Books, 1973.

Bradford, L. P. & Lippitt, R. Building a democratic work group. In G. L. Lippitt (Ed.), *Leadership in action.* Washington, D. C.: National Training Laboratories, National Education Association, 1961.

Bradford, L. P., Stock, D.. & Horwitz, M. How to diagnose group problems. In L. Bradford (Ed.), *Group development.* Washington, D.C.: National Training Laboratories, National Education Association, 1961.

Brown, E. L. Meeting patients' psychosocial needs in the general hospital. *Annals of the American Academy of Political and Social Science,* 1963, *346,* 117–125.

Brown, R. W. & Ford, M. Address in American English. *Journal of Abnormal and Social Psychology*, 1961, *62*, 375–385.

Brown, R. W. & Gilman, A. The pronouns of power and solidarity. In T. Sebeck (Ed.), *Style in language: Conference on style Indiana University, 1958*. Cambridge, Mass.: Technology Press of MIT, 1960.

Buck, R., Miller, R. E., & Caul, W. F. Sex, personality, and physiological variables in the communication of affect via facial expression. *Journal of Personality and Social Psychology*, 1974, *30*, 587–596.

Cartwright, D. & Zander, A. *Group Dynamics* (3rd Ed.). New York: Harper & Row, 1968.

Clausen, J. A. Social factors in disease. *Annals of the American Academy of Political and Social Science*, 1963, *346*, 138–148.

Coch, L., & French, J. R. P., Jr. Overcoming resistance to change. *Human Relations*, 1948, *1*, 512–532.

Cohen, M., Freedman, N., Engelhardt, D. M., & Margolis, R. A. Family interaction patterns, drug treatment and change in social aggression. *Archives of general psychiatry*, 1958, *19*, 50–56.

Cooley, C. H. *Social organization: A study of the larger mind*. New York: Scribner's, 1909.

Croog, S. H. Ethnic origins, educational level, and responses to a health questionnaire. *Human Organization*, 1961, *20*, 65–70.

Deutsch, C. P. Family factors in home adjustment of the severely disabled. *Marriage and Family Living*, 1960, *22*, 312–316.

Deutsch, M. The effects of cooperation and competition upon group processes. In D. Cartwright & A.F. Zander (Eds.), *Group dynamics: Research and theory*. Evanston, Ill.: Row, Peterson, 1953.

Deutsch, M. Conflicts: Productive and destructive (Kurt Lewin Memorial Address). *Journal of Social Issues*, 1969, *25*, 7–41.

Deutsch, M. Cooperation and trust: Some theoretical notes. In M. R. Jones (Ed.), *Nebraska Symposium on Motivation*. Lincoln: University of Nebraska Press, 1962.

Deutsch, M. & Gerard, H. B. A study of normative and informational social influences upon individual judgment. *Journal of Abnormal and Social Psychology*, 1955, *51*, 629–636.

Deutsch, M., Pepitone, A., & Zander, A. Leadership in the small group. *Journal of Social Issues*, 1948, Vol. 4.

Dewey, J. & Bentley, A. F. *Knowing and the known*. Boston: Beacon Press, 1949.

Ekman, P. Body position, facial expression and verbal behavior during interviews. *Journal of Abnormal and Social Psychology*, 1964, *68*, 295–301.

Ekman, P. Communication through non-verbal behavior: A source of information about interpersonal relations. In S. S. Tomkins & C. E. Izard (Eds.), *Affect, cognition, and personality: Empirical studies*. New York: Springer, 1965a.

Ekman, P. Differential communication of affect by head and body cues. *Journal of Personality and Social Psychology*, 1965b, *2*, 726–735.

Ekman, P. & Friesen, W. V. Detecting deception from the body or face. *Journal of Personality and Social Psychology*, 1974, *29*, 288–298.

Ekman, P., & Friesen, W. V. Non-verbal leakage and clues to deception. *Psychiatry*, 1969, *32*, 88–106.

Ekman, P., Friesen, W. V. & Ellsworth, P. *Emotion in the human face: Guidelines for research and an integration of findings.* New York: Pergamon Press, 1972.

Ellsworth, P. C. & Carlsmith, J. M. Effects of eye contact and verbal contact on affective responses to a dyadic interaction. *Journal of Personality and Social Psychology*, 1968, *10*, 15–20.

Emerson, J. Behavior in private places: Sustaining definitions of reality in gynecological examinations. In D. Brissett & C. Edgley (Eds.), *Life as theater.* Chicago: Aldine, 1975.

Ervin-Tripp, S. Sociolinguistics. In L. Berkowitz (Ed.), *Advances in experimental social psychology.* Vol. 4. New York: Academic, 1969.

Exline, R. Visual interaction: The glances of power and preference. *Nebraska Symposium on motivation*, 1971, XIX, 163–206.

Festinger, L. A theory of social comparison processes. *Human Relations*, 1954, *7*, 117–140.

Festinger L., Schachter, S., & Back, K. *Social pressures in informal groups: A study of human factors in housing.* New York: Harper, 1950.

Fielder, F. E. *A theory of leadership effectiveness.* New York: McGraw-Hill, 1967.

Freedman, N., Blass, T. Rifkin, A., & Quitkin, F. Body movements and the verbal encoding of aggressive affect. *Journal of Personality and Social Psychology*, 1973, *26*, 72–85.

Freud, S. *Collected papers.* Vols. 1–5. London: Hogarth Press, 1924–1950.

Freud, S. *Group psychology and the analysis of the ego.* New York: Bantam Books, 1960.

Garfinkel, H. *Studies in ethnomethodology.* Englewood Cliffs, N.J.: Prentice-Hall, 1967.

Gibb, C. A. Leadership. In G. Lindzey & E. Aronson (Eds.), *Handbook of social psychology* (2nd ed.). Vol. 4. Reading, Mass.: Addison-Wesley, 1969.

Glaser, B. G. & Strauss, A. L. Awareness contexts and social interaction. *American Sociology Review*, 1964, *29*, 669–679.

Goffman, E. *Frame analysis.* New York: Harper & Row, 1974.

Goffman, E. *The presentation of self in everyday life.* Garden City, N.Y.: Anchor Books, Doubleday, 1959.

Gumperz, J. J. & Hymes, D. (Eds.). *Directions in sociolinguistics.* New York: Holt, Rinehart & Winston, 1972.

Hall, E. T. Proxemics: The study of man's spatial relations. In I. Galdston (Ed.), *Man's image in medicine and anthropology: Arden House Conference on Medicine and Anthropology, 1961.* New York: International Universities Press, 1963.

Hall, E. T. *The silent language*. Garden City, N.Y.: Doubleday, 1959.

Hare, A. P. *Handbook of small group research*. Glencoe, Ill.: Free Press, 1962.

Hare, A. P. A study of interaction and consensus in different sized groups. *American Sociological Review*, 1952, *17*, 261–267.

Harlow, H. The heterosexual affectional system in monkeys. *American Psychologist*, 1962, *17*, 1–9.

Harm, C. S. & Golden, J. Group worker's role in guiding social progress in a medical institution. Social Work, 1961, *6*, 44–51.

Hollander, E. P. Conformity, status and idiosyncrasy credit. *Psychological Review*, 1958, *65*, 117–127.

Hollander, E. P. Some effects of perceived status on responses to innovative behavior. *Journal of Abnormal and Social Psychology*. 1961, *63*, 247–250.

Homans, G. C. *The human group*. New York: Harcourt, 1950.

Homans, G. C. *Social behavior: Its elementary forms*. New York: Harcourt, Brace & World, 1961.

Hyman, H. H. The psychology of status. *Archives of Psychology*, 1942, *38*, No. 269.

Hymes, D. (Ed.). *Language in culture and society: A reader in linguistics and anthropology*. New York: Harper & Row, 1964.

Hyrcenko, I. & Minton, H. L. Internal-external control, power position, and satisfaction in task-oriented groups. *Journal of Personality and Social Psychology*, 1974, *30*, 871–878.

Jackson, J. M. A space for conceptualizing person-group relationships. *Human Relations*, 159, *12*, 3–15.

Janis, I. L. Groupthink among policy makers. In N. Sanford & C. Comstock (Eds.), *Sanctions for evil*. San Francisco: Jossey-Bass, 1973.

Jones, E. E. & Gerard, H. B. *Foundations of social psychology*. New York: Wiley, 1967.

Jourard, S. M. *Disclosing man to himself*. Princeton, N.J.: Van Nostrand, 1968.

Kasl, S. V. & Mahl, G. F. The relationship of disturbances and hesitations in spontaneous speech to anxiety. *Journal of Personality and Social Psychology*, 1965, *1*, 425–433.

Kelman, H. C. Compliance, identification, and internalization: Three processes of attitude change. *Journal of Conflict Resolution*, 1958, *2*, 51–60.

Kelman, H. C. Processes of opinion change. *Public Opinion Quarterly*, 1961, *25*, 57–78.

Labov, W. *Sociolinguistic patterns*. Philadelphia: University of Pennsylvania Press, 1972.

Labov, W. *The social stratification of English in New York City*. Washington, D.C.: Center for Applied Linguistics, 1966.

Learmonth, G. J., Ackerly, W., & Kaplan, M. Relationships between palmar skin potential during stress and personality variables. *Psychosomatic Medicine*, 1959, *21*, 150–157.

Leavitt, H. J. Some effects of certain communication patterns on group performance. In E. E. Maccoby, T. M. Newcomb, & E. L. Hartley (Eds.), *Readings in social psychology* (3rd ed.). New York: Holt, 1958.

Lewin, K. *Dynamic theory of personality*. New York: McGraw-Hill, 1935.

Lewin, K. *Field theory in social science: Selected theoretical papers*, D. Cartwright (Ed.). New York: Harper & Row, 1951.

Lewin, K. Frontiers in group dynamics, I: Concept, method and reality in social science: Social equilibria and social change. *Human Relations*, 1947a, 5–41.

Lewin, K. Frontiers in group dynamics, II: Channels of group life; social planning and action research. *Human Relations*, 1947b, 143–153.

Lewin, K. Group decision and social change. In E. E. Maccoby, T. M. Newcomb, & E. L. Hartley (Eds.), *Readings in social psychology* (3rd ed.). New York: Holt, Rinehart & Winston, 1958.

Lewin, K. *Resolving social conflicts*. New York: Harper, 1948.

Lieberman, M. A., Yalom, I. D., & Miles, M. B. *Encounter groups: First facts*. New York: Basic Books, 1973.

Linton, R. *The study of man*. New York: Appleton-Century, 1936.

Lippitt, G. L. How to get results from a group. In L. P. Bradford (Ed.). *Group Development*. Washington, D.C.: National Training Laboratories, National Education Association, 1961.

Lippitt, R., & White, R. K. An experimental study of leadership and group life. In E. E. Maccoby, T. M. Newcomb, & E. L. Hartley (Eds.), *Readings in social psychology (3rd ed)*. New York: Holt, Rinehart & Winston, 1958.

Little, K. B. Cultural variations in social schemata. *Journal of Personality and Social Psychology*, 1968, *10*, 1–7.

Litwak, E. & Szelenyi, I. Primary group structures and their functions: Kin, neighbors, and friends. *American sociological review*, 1969, *34*, 465–481.

Maier, N. R. F. *Problem solving and creativity in individuals and groups*. Belmont, Calif.: Brooks/Cole, 1970.

McGregor, D. *The human side of enterprise*. New York: McGraw-Hill, 1960.

McGuire, W. J. The nature of attitudes and attitude change. In G. Lindzey & E. Aronson (Eds.), *The handbook of social psychology* (2nd ed.). Vol. 3. Reading, Mass.: Addison-Wesley, 1969.

Mead, G. H. *The social psychology of George Herbert Mead*, A. Strauss (Ed.). Chicago: University of Chicago Press, 1934.

Mechanic, D. & Volkhart, E. H. Illness behavior and medical diagnosis. *Journal of Health and Human Behavior*, 1960, *1*, 86–93.

Mehrabian, A. Nonverbal communication. *Nebraska symposium on motivation*, 1971, *XIX*, 107–162.

Merton, R. *Social theory and social structure*. (Glencoe, Ill.: Free Press, 1957.

Mills, T. M. *Group transformation*. Englewood Cliffs, N.J.: Prentice-Hall, 1964.

Moreno, J. L. *Who shall survive?* Beacon, N.Y.: Beacon House, 1953.

Moreno, J. L. *Sociometry, experimental method and the science of society*. Beacon, N.Y.: Beacon House, 1951.

Nadel, S. F. *The theory of social structure.* Glencoe, Ill.: Free Press, 1957.

Newcomb, T. M. *The acquaintance process.* New York: Holt, Rinehart & Winston, 1961.

Newcomb, T. N. Attitude development as a function of reference groups: The Bennington study. In E. E. Maccoby, T. M. Newcomb, & E. L. Hartley (Eds.), *Readings in social psychology* (3rd ed.). New York: Holt, Rinehart & Winston, 1958.

Newcomb, T. M. *Personality and social change: Attitude formation in a student community.* New York: Dryden, 1943.

Newcomb, T. M., Koenig, K. E., Flacks, R., & Warwick, D. P. *Persistance and change: Bennington College and its students after twenty-five years.* New York: Wiley, 1967.

Patterson, M. Spatial factors in social interaction. *Human Relations,* 1968, *21,* 351–361.

Porter, L. W., & Lawler, E. E. The effects of "tall" versus "flat" organization structures on managerial job satisfaction. *Personnel Psychology,* 1964, *17,* 135–148.

Raush, H. L. Interaction sequences. *Journal of Personality and Social Psychology,* 1965, *2,* 487–499.

Raven, B. H., & Rubin, J. Z. *Social Psychology: People in groups.* New York: Wiley, 1976.

Roethlisberger, F. J., Dickson, W. J., & Wright, H. A. *Management and the worker: An account of a research program conducted by the Western Electric Company, Hawthorne Works, Chicago.* Cambridge, Mass.: Harvard University Press, 1939.

Ruesch, J., & Bateson, G. *Communication: The social matrix of psychiatry.* New York: Norton, 1951.

Sampson, E. E. On justice as equality. *Journal of Social Issues,* 1975, *31,* 45–64.

Sampson, E. E. *Social psychology and contemporary society.* New York: Wiley, 1976.

Sampson, E. E. Studies of status congruence. In L. Berkowitz (Ed.), *Advances in experimental social psychology.* Vol. 4. New York: Academic Press, 1969.

Sarbin, T. R. & Allen, V. L. Role theory. In G. Lindzey & E. Aronson (Eds.), *Handbook of social psychology* (2nd ed.) Vol. 1. Reading, Mass.: Addison-Wesley, 1968.

Schachter, S. Deviation, rejection, and communication. *Journal of Abnormal and Social Psychology,* 1951, *46,* 190–207.

Scheff, T. Negotiating reality: Notes on power in the assessment of responsibility. *Social Problems,* 1968, *16,* 3–17.

Schulman, E. D. *Intervention in human services.* St. Louis: Mosby, 1974.

Schutz, A. *Collected Papers,* Vols. I–III. The Hague: Martinus Nijhoff, 1970–1971.

Schutz, W. C. *FIRO: A three-dimensional theory of interpersonal behavior.* New York: Holt, Rinehart & Winston, 1960.

Scott, T. H., Bexton, W. H., Heron, W., & Doane, B. K. Cognitive effects of perceptual isolation. *Canadian Journal of Psychology,* 1959, *13,* 200–209.

Sherif, M. A study of some social factors in perception. *Archives of Psychology,* 1935, *27,* No. 187.

Simmel, G. The number of members as determining the sociological form of the group. *American Journal of Sociology,* 1902–03, *8,* 1–46 and 158–196.

Slater, P. E. *Microcosm.* New York: Wiley, 1966.

Smith, S. L. Communication patterns and the adaptability of task-oriented groups: An experimental study. In D. Lerner & H. Lasswell (Eds.), *The policy sciences: Recent developments in scope and method.* Stanford, Calif.: Stanford University Press, 1951.

Sommer, R. *Personal space,* Englewood Cliffs, N.J.: Prentice-Hall, 1969.

Sommer, R. & Osmond, H. Symptoms of institutional care. *Social Problems,* 1960, *8,* 345–362.

Spiegel, J. *Transactions: The interplay between individual, family and society.* New York: Science House, 1971.

Spitz, R. Hospitalism: An inquiry into the genesis of psychiatric conditions in early childhood. *Psychoanalytic Study of the Child,* 1945, *1,* 53–74.

Steiger, W. A., Hoffman, F. H., Hansen, V. A., Jr., & Niebuhr, H. A definition of comprehensive medicine. *Journal of Health and Human Behavior,* 1960, *1,* 83–85.

Stock, D., Whitman, R. M., & Lieberman, M. A. The deviant member in therapy groups. *Human Relations,* 1958, *11,* 341–372.

Stogdill, R. M. Personal factors associated with leadership. *Journal of Psychology,* 1948, *25,* 35–71.

Storms, M. D. Videotape and the attribution process: Reversing actors' and observers' points of view. *Journal of Personality and Social Psychology,* 1973, *27,* 165–175.

Stouffer, S. A., Suchman, E. A., De Vinney, L. C., Star, S. A., & Williams, R. M., Jr. *The American soldier, Vol. 1. Adjustment during army life.* Princeton, N.J.: Princeton University Press, 1949a.

Stouffer, S. A., Lumsdaine, A. A., Lumsdaine, M. H., Williams, R. M., Jr., Smith, M. B., Janis, I. L., Star, S. A., & Cottrell, L. S., Jr. *The American soldier, Vol. 2. Combat and its aftermath.* Princeton: Princeton University Press, 1949b.

Strauss, A. L. *Mirrors and masks.* San Francisco: Sociology Press, 1969.

Sullivan, H. S. *The interpersonal theory of psychiatry.* New York: Norton, 1953.

Tannenbaum, R., & Schmidt, W. H. How to choose a leadership pattern. *Harvard Business Review,* 1958, *36,* 95–101.

Thelen, H. A. Work-emotionality theory of the group as organism. In S. Koch (Ed.), *Psychology: A study of a science.* Vol. 3. New York: McGraw-Hill, 1959.

Thibaut, J. W., & Kelley, H. H. *The social psychology of groups.* New York: Wiley, 1959.

Tuckman, B. W. Developmental sequence in small groups. *Psychological Bulletin,* 1965, *63,* 384–399.

Walster, E., Berscheid, E., & Walster, G. W. New directions in equity research. *Journal of Personality and Social Psychology,* 1973, *25,* 151–176.

Watzlawick, P., Beavin, J. H., & Jackson, D. D. *Pragmatics of Human Communication.* New York: Norton, 1967.

Weiss, J. Crying at the happy ending. *Psychoanalytic Review,* 1952, *39,* 388.

Weiss, J. The emergence of new themes: A contribution to the psychoanalytic theory of therapy. *International Journal of Psychoanalysis.* 1971, *52,* 459–467.

Yalom, I. D. *The theory and practice of group psychotherapy.* New York: Basic Books, 1975.

Zander, A. F., Cohen, A. R., & Stotland, E. *Role relations in the mental health professions.* Ann Arbor: Institute for Social Research, University of Michigan, 1957.

Index